C0-AZD-286

DANVILLE PUBLIC LIBRARY

3 1205 08204 8757

"Peg Jordan has done so much good behind the scenes of the health and fitness field for so many years. Her new book brings her up where she belongs . . . to the front row. Don't be left in the dark with all the new food labels. Read this book! It will light your way to healthier choices every time you shop for food!"

WITHDRAWN

Richard Simmons

"This book is on the cutting edge of nutrition education. It offers a wealth of information on interpreting the new food labels and gives the consumer solid advice on becoming one's own health advocate. A valuable resource that provides the tools to create positive lifestyle changes".

Robert Karch, Ed. D., Executive Director,
National Fitness Leaders Association, Washington, D. C.

"A win-win for consumers . . . a user-friendly book on how to read food labels and make healthy choices!"

John Cates, Executive Director,
California Governor's Council on Physical Fitness and Sports
Assistant to Arnold Schwarzenegger

". . . this book will be invaluable as a crisp, easily readable and thoroughly enjoyable guide to sound nutrition. (Jordan) is a health expert you can trust and depend on!"

Donald B. Ardell, Ph.D.
Director, *The Wellness Institute*

HOW THE
NEW FOOD LABELS
CAN SAVE YOUR
LIFE

BY PEG JORDAN, R.N.

Published by Michael Wiese Productions, 4354 Laurel
Canyon Blvd., #234, Studio City, CA 91604 (818) 379-8799.

Cover design by Art Hotel
Illustrations by Rick Stromoski

Printed by Braun-Brumfield, Inc., Ann Arbor, Michigan.
Manufactured in the United States of America.

Copyright 1994 by Michael Wiese Productions

All rights reserved. No part of this book may be reproduced
in any form or by any means without permission in writing
from the author, except for the inclusion of brief quotations
in a review.

The publisher plants two trees for every tree used in the
manufacturing of this book. Printed on recycled stock.

Library of Congress Cataloging-in-Publication Data

Jordan, Peg.
How the new food labels can save your life / by Peg Jordan
    p. cm.
Insludes bibliographical references.
ISBN 0-941188-16-7
1. Nutrition. 2. Food -- Labeling. I. Title.
RA784.J675 1992
613.2 – – dc 20   93-46754
                                                       CIP

613.2
Jor
cop.1

PUBLISHER'S NOTE

The information in this book is meant to complement the advice and guidance of your physician, not replace it. If you are under the care of a physician, you should discuss any changes in your diet with him or her.

Do not change your diet if you are seriously ill or on medication except under the care of your doctor.

The information in this book is general and should not to be taken as professional advice for your specific health problems. Any decision you make involving the treatment of an illness should include the advice of the medical doctor of your choice.

iii

"PUBLIC LIBRARY
DANVILLE, ILLINOIS"

ABOUT THE AUTHOR

Peg Jordan, R. N.

Successfully combining careers as a journalist and a registered nurse, Peg Jordan has become one of the nation's most recognized fitness writers and consumer health advocates today.

She is a frequent guest commentator for NBC's *"Today"* Show and CNN as well as the founder and editor of *American Fitness Magazine.* Ms. Jordan is a winner of the coveted *Healthy American Fitness Leader Award* from the President's Council on Physical Fitness and Sports.

Called a "health trendspotter" by *USA TODAY*, Ms. Jordan open the first hospital-based fitness center. She has written health and fitness videos for Angela Landsbury, Cher, Heather Locklear, Cathy Lee Crosby, Kathy Smith, and Richard Simmons, among others.

Ms. Jordan believes that the only way to reverse the nation's skyrocketing health care costs is by motivating and educating individuals to become their own health champions.

She resides in Pleasanton, California with her husband, four children, and two dogs.

ACKNOWLEDGMENTS

HOW THE NEW FOOD LABELS CAN SAVE YOUR LIFE
reflects the collective wisdom of the top nutritional
teachers, researchers, authors and crusading advocates
I've come to count on throughout my years of health
reporting. Those people include Michael Jacobsen,
Nancy Clark, Frank Katch, Ellen Coleman, Bonnie
Lieberman, Ann Louise Gittleman, Cheryl and Dean
Radetsky, Gail Johnston, John Travis, Lauve Metcalfe,
Sally Preston, Michael Klaper, John McDougall, Dean
Ornish and Jay Kenney.

I am indebted to Mary Beth Ferrari, my copy editor and
medical researcher, for her meticulous fact finding and
amazing wordsmith talent.

I'd like to thank Michael Wiese, a "next paradigm"
publisher whose daily brainstorms and nonstop
encouragement brought this project to fruition.

I'm also grateful to the Doctors Louis Sullivan and
David Kessler who took a courageous stand
supporting forward-thinking nutritional regulation
during a political era when regulation itself was

considered an anathema. And once the legislation was passed, I owe many thanks to Attorney Richard J. Litner, President of Nutrinfo, in Norwood., Mass., whose seminar offers valuable interpretations of the countless FDA guidelines which comprise the Nutrition Labeling and Education Act of 1990.

And finally, I'm most appreciative of my children, Claire and Adam, and my husband, Jim Kelley, who all reminded me to "stop and eat a real meal" before I grew cranky and over-hungry as I wrote this book at my computer.

TABLE OF CONTENTS

LIST OF CHARTS

INTRODUCTION

What you don't know <u>can</u> hurt you!

Saturated fats lurk in processed foods. So-called "diet" foods can be laden with animal fats. Advertising deceptively boasts of "lite" fares.

Well, dear consumer, it's time to stop swallowing pure "baloney." And it's also time to get enlightened about what really keeps you healthy.

As a health and fitness journalist, I've earned the nickname "Consumer Health Crusader" not by simply reporting medical breakthroughs (although this has merit), but also by empowering people the best way I know—with education and with the truth. These are the tools that make you the wisest health consumer you can be. And for the first time, you've got a simple-yet-powerful, little ally printed on every box of processed food. Thanks to a ten-year, concerted effort by private action groups, public information councils and government agencies, we have one of the most enlightened tools for dietary health—the new nutrition label.

I wrote this book to share with you what I've learned about the label, its advantages, its short-comings and how to use it to calculate—and consume—a healthy diet.

So here's to saving your life!

Peg Jordan, R.N.

1

READ THIS BOOK—
AND SAVE YOUR LIFE!

Reading a book on food labels to "save your life" may sound a bit outrageous, but that claim is based on a startling new finding that science recently uncovered. And since that finding has everything to do with **you and your food choices**, it's high time you were **informed** about it! The top researchers in the country, recognized health professionals—even the U.S. Department of Health and Human Services—know beyond a doubt that **the typical American diet is basically killing us**.

The leading causes of death for most Americans— heart disease and certain cancers—are preventable! And five of the top ten causes are all diet-related. That's right—**you can prevent** the current chief killers from ruining your life and the lives of your loved ones by changing your food choices. Now be prepared: you're going to read that more than once in this book, because I find that it takes people a while to really let that message sink in.

3

If you want to enjoy a healthy life, you must pay attention to what you eat. The development of the new and improved labels is chiefly the result of "a clear and crucial connection between diet and health." That's according to Louis W. Sullivan, M.D., a former Secretary of Health and Human Services and an important player in the campaign to implement the labeling changes. By using the information on the new labels wisely, you have the ability and information to wipe out the number one killers, and you can also reduce the threat of other related "diseases of lifestyle"—namely, obesity, high blood pressure, arthritis, adult onset diabetes, osteoporosis, gastrointestinal ailments and more.

So, once again, hear it loud and clear. You have the resources today to wipe out the possibility of chronic, degenerative, life-threatening disease and premature death. It's well within your grasp.

In fact, it's right at your fingertips.

Eliminating the Mystery

This is what *How the New Food Labels Can Save Your Life* explores. With everything the medical profession has proven about disease prevention and health promotion, it's pure insanity to not take advantage of that knowledge and arm ourselves with all the facts necessary to ensure good health. With the right information and committed action, you can start to eat better, and:

- Enjoy vibrant, good health and increased energy,
- Reach/maintain your healthy weight naturally, and
- Increase your life span.

One of the easiest ways to take control of your health is by taking the mystery out of the food selection process. That's what the new food label can do for you. Reading it can help you navigate around the nutritional booby traps hidden on supermarket shelves. At a press conference given on the new food labels, Sullivan, then Secretary of Health and Human Services, specified exactly what the new food labels will do. We will all benefit, he promised, from labels that:

- Communicate more information intelligently to the consumer;

- Make a difference in the ability of consumers to make informed choices about the nutritional value of foods they buy;

- Ensure that those choices can be made with the full confidence that the information on the label is reliable and based on scientific fact—not advertising or marketing hype; and perhaps most importantly,

- Give consumers the power to take an active, responsible role in protecting and promoting their health.

With this new label, we have moved directly to the supermarket shelf with the information consumers need to select healthier diets. Before the new food label was developed, people really didn't know how to correctly evaluate the saturated fats, cholesterol and other undesirables lurking in packaged and processed foods without resorting to higher mathematics, carrying around a brand-name list compiled by public interest groups, and calculating the real truth behind the hype. How to separate the healthy foods from those that deserve a warning label basically remained a mystery—and the consumer remained in the dark.

Remember, it's always been a "buyer-beware" market out there. That's why I'm pushing a new motto: "buyer-be-educated." The sole purpose of the food industry is to sell products, not to teach you about the healthiest choices. It's far easier to manufacture a microwave dinner with cheap sources of saturated fats, and sell it through deceptive advertising messages, such as "lite!" and "Less fat!" than to manufacture it with the costlier, non-fat items that are far healthier.

Over the years, legions of consumers grew dissatisfied with inadequate food labels, and not only with the deceptive ones. Scores of different food products had no label at all. Some labels featured a few ingredients but failed to include the more disastrous items. Today, with the new label, all that has changed. Now you've got a means for deciphering the mystery. Reading labels is the easiest, most effective way to increase your awareness about healthy and not-so-healthy foods.

Why Do We Need a "Nutrition Facts" Label?

If it's just a matter of knowing what's healthy and what's not, why do we really need a new food label? Good question. Many folks believe that there is already too much government regulation, and that big brother shouldn't demand that the food industry spend $2 billion to relabel packages. But others, such as consumer advocates, justifiably argue that no matter what the initial cost is for relabeling, we will no doubt save billions more in reduced health costs from improved nutrition.

Well, I stand with the consumer advocates. We have more research literature than ever that documents a connection between diet and the risk of disease. Plus, we've also got a skyrocketing national health bill, ready to top $900 billion annually! While everybody screams for health care reform, the real action can start with you. The last three Surgeon Generals have all agreed: *prevention* is the name of the game if we're to cure our sickly national health debt and wipe out our chief killers today—heart disease, stroke and certain cancers. And everybody knows—prevention starts with an apple a day. So, it's time to read the label, Mabel.

You've seen the new label format on some food items since the spring of 1993. As a result of the passage of the Nutrition Labeling and Education Act, the redesigned label must be present on all processed foods regulated by the Food and Drug Administration by May 1994. The sooner you understand the labels, the better you will fare.

Couldn't I Just Determine a Healthy Diet All on My Own?

Sure. You're smart enough to determine the make-up of a healthy diet. But do you really know what constitutes 30 grams of fat in a daily menu? Most experts wouldn't know without a label. And more importantly, have you ever been influenced by advertising? You bet you have. Since about the age of two. Want some proof? What if I started singing, "You deserve a break today at..." You just finished the jingle, didn't you? And how about: "Trix are for ...." See what I mean?

Advertising hype in the food industry is perhaps the most pervasive, hard-hitting, non-stop pounding out there. Words such as "lite," "reduced," "cholesterol free," "fiber rich," are everywhere. When you pick up a package of hot dogs hyping "85% fat free," do you realize they're basing this on weight and not the actual nutritional value? You may be lured into buying something that is actually 60% fat—just because of a misleading label. (More on this later.)

Government Intervention

Let's take a moment to consider the history of progress in food labeling. In 1938, the Food and Drug Administration issued regulations stipulating that all packaged foods had to carry a label that gave the product, name and location of the manufacturer, packer or distributor and the net content or weight in pounds or fluid ounces. Beyond those basics, food labels were largely a defensive strategy.

Manufacturers used them to tell shoppers that foods were free of harmful substances.

Then, in 1973, the government adopted a protective stance and began to use labels to provide nutritional information in the form of listings of calories, vitamins and minerals to aid meal planners. In effect, the labels said, "These nutritional elements are present to this degree in this product." The food labels were also required to list ingredients by specific name, in descending order of weight. Though only twenty years have passed, the food labeling implemented in 1973 has already become obsolete.

The new labels take us another leap forward. After years of debate and lots of long-winded speeches about the beauty of the free market system, our government is just now getting around to giving us the straight scoop about the food we eat. Well, actually we're not getting a full education, but we are getting a revolutionary new food label, and—rumor has it—an education program that will teach us how to use it.

Welcome to the Nutrition Labeling and Education Act of 1990 (NLEA). This system of mandatory nutrition labeling for foods takes one giant step forward in the direction of making food labeling information consistent with recent dietary recommendations from the U.S. Surgeon General and the National Research Council. As a consumer, you will receive many exciting benefits from this dramatically new nutrition labeling.

Today, many of us are getting more than we need of the essential nutrients listed on the old labels. We are getting so much of some nutrients—fat, for example—that we are endangering our health. Cancer, stroke, diabetes and atherosclerosis account for approximately 68% of deaths annually in our country. Government health officials estimate that between 50% and 80% of these early deaths might be prevented through proper diet.

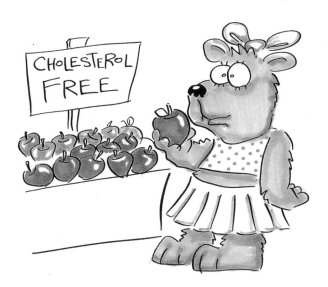

It's not that you need a degree to read and interpret the new food labels, but they do present some unique challenges for the average consumer. Word is the government plans to follow the advice of our old friend, Ruskin, and provide the public with an educational program to explain the labels and their use. But since that program is only in the planning stages and is rumored to have a small budget, you've done yourself a favor by purchasing this book.

Learning to read and understand the nutrition facts in the new food labels will help you to make healthy food choices. And since five of the leading causes of death in our country—heart disease, stroke, cancer, diabetes and chronic liver disease/cirrhosis —are diet-related to some degree, what you will learn in these pages can directly affect your health. Reading this book will definitely save you time in the grocery store, but more importantly using what you learn here can prolong your life!

> *We used to get diseases of deficiencies.*
> *Now we get diseases of excess.*
> *The old label said,*
> *"Make sure you get enough nutrients, honey."*
> *The new labels says,*
> *"Hold off, partner, aren't you at your limit?"*

THE NEW FOOD LABEL– WHAT IT WILL DO

It was not an easy birth. There were more than two years of discussion and deliberation about the new food labels. In fact, development and resolution were moving so slowly that the American Heart Association threatened a lawsuit. Finally in December of 1992, the Bush Administration approved legislation — the Nutrition Labeling and Education Act—authorizing the most extensive food labeling reform in the history of this country.

As a result, food manufacturers have until May 1994 to implement labeling changes. You've already seen the new label format on some food items. Other food manufacturers have requested and obtained extensions of time for compliance with the new labeling regulations. There will be delays, as there always are when change occurs, but eventually use of this revolutionary nutritional aid will be widespread enough to offer several potential health benefits.

Read the Directions!

What's the first thing you should do after you purchase a new product or device? That's right—

read the directions. You derive the greatest benefit
from any product if you know how to operate or
use it in the way that it was designed to be used.
The same fact is true of the new food labels. These
nutrition panels won't solve all your dietary
dilemmas, but the information they contain will
enable you to make wiser food choices and,
therefore, decrease your risk of disease. But the
labels can only help you accomplish these goals *if*
you know how to read and interpret the
information they provide.

In order to make certain you understand the new
lables, we're going to study a sample label one
section at a time. So, follow along. You'll be
surprised—and pleased—at what you learn.

PRESENTING.... THE NEW LABEL

NUTRITION FACTS	
Serving Size 2 ounces	
Servings Per Container 6	

Amount Per Serving	
Calories 220	Calories from Fat 27

	% Daily Value *
Total Fat 3 g	5 %
Saturated Fat 0.5 g	2 %
Cholesterol 54 mg	20 %
Sodium 28 mg	1.2%
Total Carbohydrate 40 g	13 %
Dietary Fiber 0 g	-
Sugars 1 g	-
Protein 8 g	-

* Percent Daily values are based on a 2000 calorie diet. Your daily values may be higher or lower depending on your calorie needs:

	Calories	2000	2500
Total Fat	Less than	65 g	80 g
Sat Fat	Less than	20 g	25 g
Cholesterol	Less than	300 mg	300 mg
Sodium	Less than	2400 mg	2400 mg
Total Carbohydrate		300 g	375 g
Dietary Fiber		25 g	30 g

Calories per gram:

Fat 9	•	Carbohydrate 4	•	Protein 4

Start With Servings

Immediately under the bold new heading of
Nutrition Facts is information you will recognize:
Serving Size and **Servings Per Container.**
"Nothing new here," you say. "Food labels have
always given these figures, at least in my lifetime."
But, look again. There is a difference. In the old
days of labeling, serving sizes were not regulated, so
food manufacturers were able to practice the high
art of illusion. For instance, suppose a food product
was quite high in calories and fat content. One way
for a manufacturer to create the illusion of fewer
calories and less fat was to reduce the serving size.

You've had the experience I'm sure. You conscien-
tiously scan the calorie and fat content for one
serving before purchasing your favorite frozen
yogurt and feel positively gleeful. It seems too
good to be true: the taste of ice cream for the
calorie cost of jello. That is until you figured out
that the only person who would be satisfied with
such a minuscule serving was your two-year-old
nephew.

This sad little scenario will be brought to a just end
by new regulations which insist that manufacturers
conform to a standard serving size, one that is more
in line with what people really eat. **Serving Size,**

Servings Per Container and then **Calories Per Serving** will be realistic and meaningful figures on the new food label—figures that are based on food consumption surveys that reflect amounts people actually consume. For example, the standard serving size for cookies will be 30 grams. "So what's a gram?" you say. "And how do I know when I have 30 of them?"

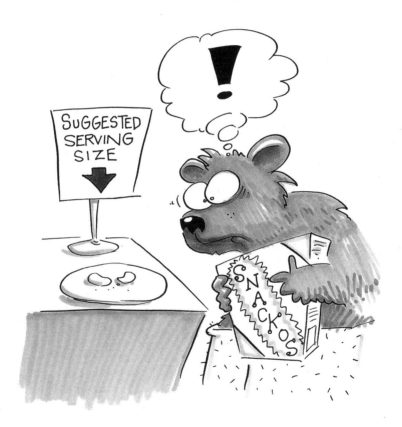

Never fear... Those Keebler elves and all the others responsible for the convoys of cookies in our markets must list exactly how many cookies comprise 30 grams.

You see how it works? The new labels will not make your eyes glaze over with never-ending lists of vitamins and minerals, but they will make you think and that's the idea. Think and plan and choose wisely. The labels give you the information you need to put together a healthful diet. All you have to do is use it.

Fat Is the Villain

Right up front and directly across **Calories** (per serving) is a new figure: **Calories from Fat,** the real dietary culprits according to nutritionists nationwide. The experts whose job it is to tell us how to eat in order to enjoy good health say we should get no more than 30% of our daily calories from fat. Some authorities insist that figure is too high, that fat calories should account for no more than 20% or even 10% of our diets. I recommend working toward the lower percentages of 20 or 10%. Whichever percentage you aim for, the real point is that the new food labels will help you plan a program and stick to it.

Next on the label is a listing of nutrients that are important to the good health of Americans *today*. Many of us are getting more than we need of the essential nutrients listed on the old labels. In fact, many experts feel that rather than being a country that is not getting enough vitamins and minerals, we are a country suffering from the problems of overconsumption. For example, most Americans consume more than twice the amount of protein required for health maintenance. Our concern is not with nutritional deficiencies. What we really lack—and what the new labels provide—is an *understanding* of how certain important nutrients contribute to a healthful diet, and ultimately, a healthier body.

On the left side of the label under the heading **Amount Per Serving** and directly below the number of calories is a straightforward listing (in grams) of **Total Fat, Saturated Fat, Cholesterol, Sodium, Total Carbohydrate, Dietary Fiber, Sugars, Protein, Vitamin A, Vitamin C, Iron** and **Calcium**. Each listing represents the amount of a particular nutrient supplied by a single serving, expressed in grams (g.) or milligrams (mg.). With this information, you can compare food products and keep track of how much of each nutrient you are consuming as the day progresses.

Lose the Fat

For the first time in history, food labels will tell us not only how many grams of **Total Fat** are present (including monounsaturated, polyunsaturated and saturated fat) but also how many of those grams are **Saturated Fat**. Here is information that is absolutely essential to the planning of a healthful diet. Why? Because although the government is telling us that calories from fat should account for no more than 30% of our daily caloric intake, it is also telling us that only one-third of those fat calories should be from saturated fat—the villain responsible for clogging arteries and increasing the risk of heart disease.

Additional help for your heart is contained in the **Cholesterol** count per serving which appears next in milligrams. Because certain kinds of cholesterol clog arteries and contribute to heart disease, this figure is one to note carefully as you consult a product's label.

The amount of **Sodium** per serving is also listed in milligrams. Since sodium is a contributing factor in hypertension and heart disease, a wise shopper will pay attention to how much is present.

The number of grams of **Total Carbohydrate** that is furnished in one serving is the next listing on the label, followed by the grams of **Sugars** and **Dietary Fiber**. Carbohydrate sources include simple sugars and complex carbohydrates (starches and fibers). Most foods contain a combination of these carbohydrate sources, so careful consideration of these numbers is recommended. A diet that favors complex carbohydrates will generally provide more vitamins, minerals and fiber for the calorie cost than a diet that emphasizes sugars.

Knowing how much simple sugar is present in one serving is information that is crucial for diabetics and hypoglycemics. We all profit from knowing how much dietary fiber a food product contains since fiber helps to prevent cancer and heart disease. **Most Americans get less than half of the fiber they need each day.** Because fiber content is listed on the new label, you will have an easier time choosing foods that are fiber rich.

Protein is the final nutrient listed in total grams per serving. Since proteins contain amino acids which are the body's building blocks, essential to the growth and repair of tissues, enzymes, hormones, antibodies and blood cells, this is an important figure for everyone to consider when making a food choice.

% Daily Value

The next section of the label is fascinating to me in terms of the information it gives. On the right and corresponding to the amount of each nutrient supplied by a single serving is a new number called the **% Daily Value**. And this is the smart part. Simply put, **% Daily Value** shows how a food fits into your daily diet. Not so simply put, the new label will tell you not only how many grams of, let's say, dietary fiber are in that bagel you are contemplating but also *how much that serving will contribute toward your total daily intake of dietary fiber* (**% Daily Value**).

Let's say the bagel has three grams of dietary fiber. That would make its Daily Value 12%, meaning 12% of the recommended maximum daily intake for that nutrient. Eating that bagel will give you 12% of the dietary fiber you need for the day. Now all you have to do is make food choices that will give you the remaining 88% of your fiber requirement for that day. I'm impressed! Here is the government supplying us with information *and* education. Let's try another example: If the glass of cranberry juice you had with your breakfast accounted for 60% of your vitamin C requirement for the day, then you're in pretty good shape. One medium-sized apple, and you've probably reached your quota of Vitamin C until tomorrow. If you want to make absolutely certain you've gotten all the Vitamin C you need, be sure to finish at least one serving of broccoli at dinner.

One of the most important pieces of information provided in the % Daily Value column is what percentage of your daily fat intake each food contains. This is based on the goal of 30% fat per day which can also be expressed as 65 grams of fat for a 2000 a day diet.

Here's an example. Let's say you know from past label scans that the snack food you are contemplating contains only 3 grams of fat per serving. The *new* food label takes one giant, positive step forward and tells you that these 3 grams of fat constitute only 5% of your day's fat allowance. Aim for daily value percentages for fat that are around or below 5% because they will add up fast throughout the day. The U.S. Department of Agriculture has determined that the average person eats about 20 food items a day. If each contains about 5% of your allotted fat intake for the day, you'll be right on target. Selecting items that are 5% or less will make room for a few items that may be a little higher.

Nutrition experts nationwide have determined what amounts constitute 100% of the fat, saturated fat, cholesterol, sodium, carbohydrate and fiber that should be consumed each day. The numbers in the **% Daily Value** column represent the percentage of that nutrient that is contributed by one serving of the food whose label you are consulting.

The Percent Daily Value figures are based on a 2000 calorie diet, the daily calorie consumption of the "average" person. "But, I'm not average," you say. "If I ate 2000 calories a day, I'd gain weight!" Or, perhaps your problem is just the opposite, and you need *more* than 2000 calories to make it through the day. You can still use these Daily Values as guides.

Why? One reason is that the Daily Values for sodium and cholesterol are the same for everyone regardless of the number of calories consumed. Another reason is that The National Academy of Sciences recommends that all healthy adults consume no more than 2400 milligrams of sodium daily. And no matter what your height or weight, the National Cholesterol Education Program recommends no more than 300 milligrams of cholesterol.

Finally, the Daily Values for vitamins and minerals are based on the U.S. Recommended Daily Allowances for each specific nutrient. These allowances are uniform for all and are not based on any particular calorie count.

So, when it comes to sodium, cholesterol, vitamins and minerals, daily allowances are standard. That means you can take the figure in the **% Daily Value** column at face value. If the prepared pasta dish you are planning for dinner supplies 28% of your sodium intake for the day, it provides approximately the same percentage for your wife or your husband or your neighbor next door.

On the other hand, for fat, saturated fat, total carbohydrates, dietary fiber and protein, you might have to do some simple calculations. This is because daily values for these nutrients *will* fluctuate depending upon the number of calories an individual consumes. As I mentioned earlier, the government is recommending that fat calories account for no more than 30% of your total calorie count each day, and is further advising that saturated fat calories be no more than 10%. Nutritionists consistently recommend that at least 60% of your daily calorie total come from carbohydrates and that you provide about 11.5 grams of fiber for every 1000 calories you take in. Finally, if as little as 10% of your total calories are provided by protein sources, your need for this important nutrient will have been met. It doesn't take a calculator to see that most of us exceed this need on a pretty regular basis.

The truth is that the percentages in the **Daily Value** column can still serve as guides, no matter what your size or calorie intake. If you eat more than 2000 calories a day, you know you can afford a little more of the food in question. If your diet consists of fewer than 2000 calories a day, you must adjust your intake accordingly.

One of the greatest advantages of the **% Daily Value** figures is that they will enable you to compare food products and make rational choices. For example, on a recent visit to my neighborhood supermarket, I literally talked a woman out of purchasing a chicken pie that would have used up a whopping 32 grams (or more than 50%) of her daily fat allowance! Instead, I directed her to the end of the aisle where free samples of a prepared vegetarian pizza were being distributed. Total fat for the entire pizza which combined vitamin C-rich veggies and a low-fat cheese? Only 8 grams or approximately 15% of her Daily Value. A much better deal for her heart and her overall health. Once you've read this book, you'll be able to do the same thing for yourself.

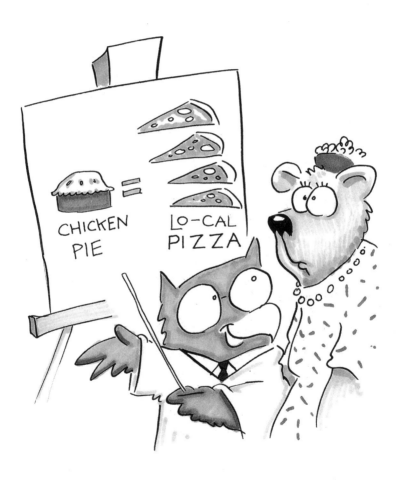

In addition to values for the nutrients above, the new food labels will list the % **Daily Values** for four additional and essential nutrients: vitamin A, vitamin C, calcium and iron.

Health Claims

One of the most dramatic differences between the new labels and the old is that the new format may include a health claim—if it is relevant. In seven very specific situations, a manufacturer may call attention to the connection between a particular food or nutrient and a reduced risk of a certain disease, an action that was forbidden by law prior to the NLEA.

The seven nutrient/disease relationships are:

- Calcium and osteoporosis;

- Fat and cancer;

- Saturated fat, cholesterol and coronary heart disease;

- Fiber-containing grain products, fruits and vegetables, and cancer;

- Fruits, vegetables, and grain products that contain fiber, and coronary heart disease;

- Sodium and high blood pressure; and

- Fruits, vegetables and cancer.

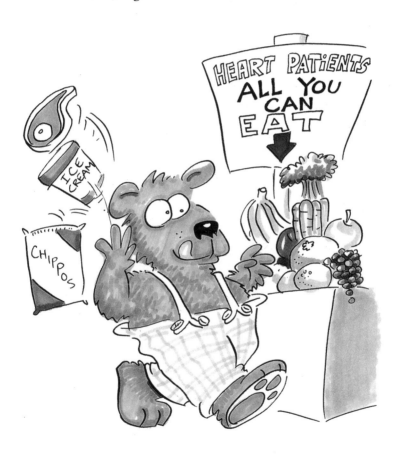

29

"PUBLIC LIBRARY DANVILLE, ILLINOIS"

Because scientific evidence of the link between food and disease has increased tremendously in the past decade, claims for the specific relationships cited above may be included on food labels using statements, symbols or descriptions.

As you might expect, the rules concerning the use of health claims are very strict. For example, the juice manufacturer who has added calcium can only claim (on the label) that the product "may" or "might" reduce osteoporosis. And, in order to legally make this claim, the calcium must be present in a form that is easily absorbed. What's more, the label must contain a statement that acknowledges that other factors play a part in the risk reduction. For example, calcium *and* sufficient weight-bearing exercise *may* reduce the risk of osteoporosis.

So, look for these claims on the new food labels. Consider them prudently and remember it's a "may" or "might" situation we're talking about here. But "may" or "might" is better than not at all. If you are concerned about any of the illnesses or conditions cited above, you would be wise to consider foods and nutrients that promise a reduction of risk.

"Less" Is More

One of the most refreshing and constructive changes to occur as a result of the NLEA is the development of specific definitions for such nutritional marketing terms as "light" and "low fat." Manufacturers may only use the following terms if their products truly fit the bill:

- **Free** - This description may be used on packaging only if a product contains none or negligible amounts of fat, saturated fat, cholesterol, sodium, sugar and/or calories.

- **Good Source** - If one serving of the food supplies between 10 and 19% of the Daily Value for a specific nutrient, the food can be considered a "good source."

- **High** - When a single serving of the food in question contains at least 20% or more of the Daily Value for a particular nutrient, this descriptive term may apply.

- **Lean** and **Extra Lean** - are used to describe the fat content of certain meats, poultry, seafood and game meats.

Lean can be used if less than 10 grams of fat, less than 4 grams of saturated fat, and less than 95 milligrams of cholesterol are present per serving.

Extra Lean is reserved for fat contents of fewer than 5 grams, with less than 2 grams of saturated fat, and fewer than 95 milligrams of cholesterol per serving.

• **Less** - If a food contains 25% *less* of a particular nutrient than a comparable food, this description can be used. The word *Fewer* can be used in the same situation.

• **Light** - has more than one meaning, so buyer beware!

Light may mean that a food has been nutritionally altered so as to contain at least one third less calories than its original counterpart, or

Light may mean that a food's fat content has been lessened by at least one-half. In fact, a food that contains 50% or more of its calories from fat must reduce its fat content by at least one-half in order to be dubbed *light*, but...

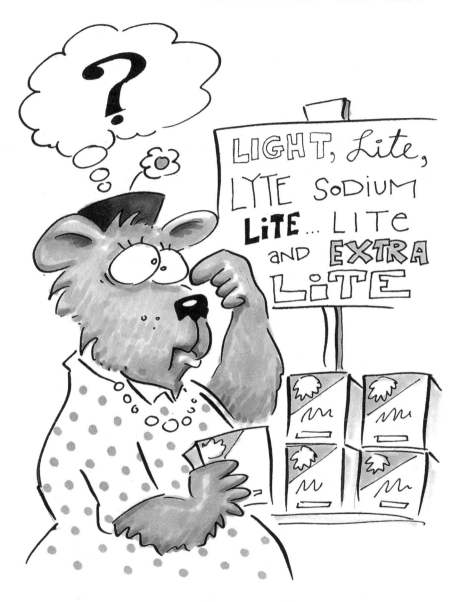

Light is also used to signify that the sodium content of a low-calorie, low-fat food has been reduced by at least 50%. And if the food is not low in fat and calories and the sodium level has been reduced by one-half, the label must read *Light in Sodium.* Finally,

Light can legitimately be used to describe an entire meal or main dish that is low in fat or calories. And as always,

Light will continue to be used quite aptly to describe texture or color. But, the label must be specific so that its meaning is clear. For example, because its spelled out, we understand that *light brown sugar* means sugar that is pale brown in color, not low in calories.

• **Low** - is another description that may require some homework. Basically, if a person can eat a food frequently without exceeding dietary guidelines for fat, saturated fat, cholesterol, sodium, and/or calories, the food in question may be considered *low.* You don't have to be a scientist to think that this cannot be the whole story, and you're right. You owe yourself at least a nodding acquaintance with the details:

Low Fat means a food has a fat content of 3 grams or less per serving.

Low Saturated Fat is reserved for foods that contain no more than 1 gram of this culprit per serving.

Low Sodium can only be used if 100 grams of the food contains 140 milligrams or less of sodium.

Very Low Sodium signifies an extremely low level of this nutrient—no more than 35 milligrams per serving.

Low Cholesterol means a single serving (approximately 100 grams) contains less than 20 milligrams.

Low Calorie is restricted to food products that have 40 calories or less in one serving. It may also be used to describe entire meals, such as frozen dinners, that contain 120 calories or less per 100 grams (about 3.5 ounces).

• **More** - on a food label tells you that a product contains at least 10% more of the Daily Value for a particular nutrient than its original counterpart. The next time your favorite cereal or yogurt claims to be calcium-fortified, check it out.

- **Reduced** - This is a tricky one. If a food product has been nutritionally altered and contains 25% less of a specific nutrient or 25% fewer calories than the original, it can legitimately be called *Reduced*. However, if the original product were *Low* in a particular nutrient, the quantity of that nutrient cannot be additionally lessened, and the product, therefore, termed *Reduced*. Did you follow that? Let's say that I manufacture a luscious, but low-calorie new dessert that has the requisite 40 calories or fewer per serving. I cannot fiddle with this new find, lessen the calorie count still further, and call it *Reduced*. Those are the rules.

- **Percent Fat Free** - This phrase is usually accompanied by a number. For example, the packaging for one brand of turkey hot dogs now sports a banner that loudly proclaims: *85% fat free!* What does it mean? In this case, the eye-catching phrase means that 85% of the *weight* of each hot dog is fat free. One serving or one hot dog weighs 45 grams. Only 7 of those grams are fat grams. That leaves 38 grams which can legally be called fat free!

But that's not all there is to it. Notice that I have emphasized the word *weight*. It is, after all, the key word in the equation because—stay with me now— **98% fat free by weight is not the same as 98%**

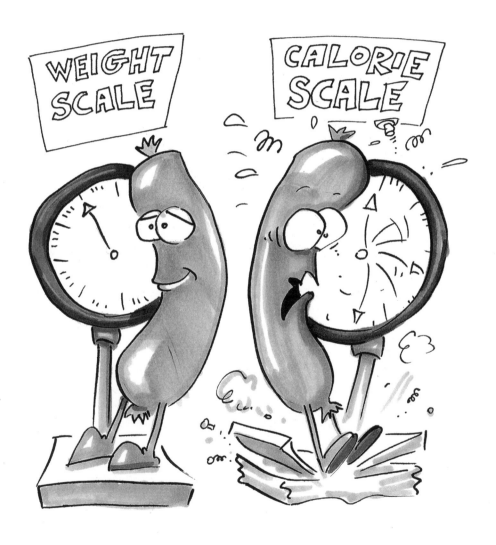

fat free by calories. To illustrate, let's go back to the turkey franks. Say that each hot dog has 90 calories. Remember that I mentioned that each hot dog has 7 grams of fat. Now each individual gram of fat always equals 9 calories. So we multiply the number of grams (7) by the number of calories (9), and see that a total of 63 calories in each hot dog are fat calories (9 x 7 = 63). From here, it's a small leap to the realization that the hot dogs may be 85% fat free by weight, but they are certainly not 85% fat free by calories. In truth, these franks get approximately 70% of their calories from fat! So, be careful. Once I figured out this mind bender, I began a search for a more authentically low-fat lunch alternative to turkey hot dogs.

• **Implied Claims** - Finally, we have protection against statements whose main purpose seems to be to mislead, confound and confuse. They are simply not allowed under the new labeling law. For example, if a muffin manufacturer wants to be able to bill his bakery products as *Made with Oat Bran*, he must see that they contain enough oat bran to meet the definition requirements for *a good source of fiber* (one serving = 10-19% of Daily Value for fiber). Similarly, a product may not brag *No Tropical Oils* unless it is truly low in *all* saturated fats.

These regulations offer welcome relief to the dishonest labeling practices of the past.

Specifics Satisfy

Today's food labels are new and improved in many
ways, not the least of which is more conscientious
attention to detail. "Oh no," you say, "that
probably means the labels will be longer and harder
to read." Not true. What it really means is that
you will finally get enough information to know the
truth.

For example, no longer will a manufacturer be able
to state simply that a food product contains *colors*.
All color additives must be specified by name. This
is good news for those who suffer from allergies or
sensitivities to such substances. If you can see that a
food contains an additive that causes you trouble,
you can just cross it off your grocery list.

Here's one I love. I'm certain you encountered the
word *flavorings* on the old food labels. Or sometimes it was *other flavorings*. Usually the phrase was
found as the final item in a long, long list of ingredients for such items as salad dressing. It always
seemed as though the manufacturer just kind of ran
out of steam and didn't feel like taking the trouble
to list the flavorings by name, whatever they were.
I don't know about you, but it did leave me with a
strange kind of label anxiety. It was a catch-all, it's-
anybody's-guess kind of term. Who knew what

flavorings meant? Not I, that's for sure. And, I'll bet you didn't either. Well, we no longer have to worry. It seems that these mysterious ingredients are generally sources of protein hydrolysates, many of which are high in sodium. As such, they must now be listed by name so they can be recognized by people who must follow low-sodium diets.

And it's curtains for my personal favorite—the juice scam. How many times have you purchased a juice drink only to get it home and discover that it contains a wide variety of ingredients, but precious little of the fruit juice you were craving and thought you were buying. That can't happen any more because manufacturers must state the exact percentage of juice that is contained in the drink. And if a manufacturer has combined small amounts of several different types of juice into one drink, special restrictions apply. Let's say that blueberry, apple and pear juices have been combined The resulting beverage cannot be called *blueberry juice* even if that juice is present in a larger quantity than the other two. The manufacturer must name the drink more accurately, such as *blueberry-flavored juice drink* or state the amount of blueberry juice present within 5% of the actual amount.

So, there you have it: Truth in Labeling—at last. **The new label is the first federally approved**

food label that actually links daily diet to good health. The information contained in the new labels is there to help you protect your health from the chronic problems that have plagued generations of Americans.

One Size Does Not Really Fit All

Just a few pointers before we move on. It is wise to keep in mind, as mentioned earlier, that the FDA has based the ideal daily intakes for fat, carbohydrates and other nutrients on a daily diet of 2000 calories. Thus, we are working with specific recommended quantities: 65 grams or less of fat, 20 grams or less of saturated fat, 300 milligrams or less of cholesterol, 2400 milligrams or less of sodium, at least 300 grams of carbohydrates, and 25 grams of fiber. Ideal amounts for sugar and protein were not determined.

RECOMMENDED DAILY QUANTITIES
FOR FAT, CARBOHYDRATES, SODIUM AND FIBER
FOR A 2000 CALORIE DIET

FAT	65 grams or less
SATURATED FAT	20 grams or less
CHOLESTEROL	300 milligrams or less
SODIUM	2400 milligrams or less
CARBOHYDRATES	at least 300 grams
FIBER	25 grams

Amounts selected by the Food and Drug Administration.
Recommendations for sugar and protein were not determined.

The reality is that the **recommended daily calorie amounts vary depending upon the individual.** Most men consume somewhat more than 2000 calories a day, perhaps as many as 2500. Women, on the other hand, seem to fare quite well with somewhere between 1900 and 2200 calories. As you might expect, important differences show up in the resulting recommendations for important nutrients. For example, the FDA believes that women should consume no more than 65 grams of fat in a day, while men are considered safe with an intake of up to 80 grams. Finally, we have people with special calorie needs: children, the elderly, athletes.

As a compromise, a third panel was added to the bottom of the new label. This section lists the FDA's guidelines by weight for both a 2000 and 2500 calorie diet. If you consume 2000 calories a day, you'll have no trouble finding accurate percentages in the % **Daily Values** column as explained earlier. But, if you eat 2500 calories a day, you'll have to do a little work to figure out the percentages of recommended nutrients in one serving of a particular food.

As a test case, let's suppose you are considering a purchase of macaroni and cheese for dinner. Your doctor has told you to go easy on fat, and you know that cheese is a rich source of fat. You'd like to have some idea what this choice will do to your fat intake for the day, before you plunk your money down. The label says that one serving, which equals one-half a cup, contains 13 grams of fat. All you have to do is to divide the 13 grams by the 80 grams per day of fat listed under the 2500 calorie heading, and you'll find that one serving of this main dish will provide approximately 16% of your daily recommended fat intake. It's that simple, and you can use the same formula for any nutrient on the label. **Divide and Conquer!**

To figure out how much fat a particular food contributes to your overall fat intake, remember this simple formula.

FORMULA TO CALCULATE
% DAILY VALUE FOR FAT

Number of Fat Grams Listed Per Serving	*Divided By*	Total Daily Intake of Fat Listed for Calorie Category (2000 or 2500)	Equals	% of Your Recommended Fat Intake the Serving
Contains				

"Oh great," you say. "As if I don't have enough to do. I'll just spend my days wandering up and down supermarket aisles with a slide rule and a calculator." Not so. The truth is, once you've done a few of these calculations, you'll get the hang of it and be able to estimate in many cases. After all, a percentage or two in one direction or another is not going to ruin your diet or your health. The real point is that you are headed in the right direction. Also, once you've figured the percentage of fat one serving of macaroni and cheese contributes to your daily diet, you'll remember it for next time. You may not recall the specific numbers, but you'll probably remember whether the food is worth the cost of the fat. The question is: Can you afford it?

So gradually you won't be doing a lot of figuring and calculating. You will learn over time that you can afford to eat certain foods while others are simply too costly for your nutritional budget.

THE NEW FOOD LABEL— WHAT IT WON'T DO

My cousin Louie is the family philosopher. He likes to say that nothing in life is 100%. What he means is that nothing is perfect, an observation that is certainly true of the new food labels.

The new labels give us a lot of very important and useful information. However, there are some facts that are simply not provided, and, believe it or not, there are also some leftover shady areas that will successfully confuse or mislead the consumer who is not careful. I'll explain.

The Lunchtime Lesson

Remember the lesson of the turkey hot dogs that I shared with you in the last chapter? It's one that warrants a brief review: The brand in question boasts newly designed packaging that proudly displays the following marketing magic: *85% Fat Free, 15% Fat*. I was taken in at first as I'm certain most consumers are. The problem, if you recall, is that the catchy phrase refers to percent fat by weight, not percent fat by calories. And, the difference that distinction makes is significant.

45

Just watch. One turkey frank or "link" (as the manufacturer calls it) weighs 45 grams. Of those 45 grams, 7 grams are from fat. Thus, the 15% fat figure that is cited on the label. When it comes to calories, however, the story is dramatically different. Each link equals 90 calories. Since, one gram of fat has 9 calories, we multiply 7 (the grams of fat in one frank) by 9 (the calories in one gram of fat) for a grand total of 63. In other words, 63 of the 90 calories in one frank are calories from fat. I'm no wizard when it comes to math, but even I can see at a glance that each turkey hot dog is approximately 70% fat! Not the best choice for a low fat lunch.

How can this happen, you ask? Nutrition claims such as *Percent Fat Free* are precisely defined under the Food and Drug Administration's new rules. The problem is that **processed meats like hot dogs are not regulated** by the FDA, so confusing claims like this one can still pop up to mislead you.

The Sugar Free Story

Under the new labeling regulations, *sugar free* means less than 0.5 grams of sugar per serving. The positive sounding phrase has become a popular one and is used frequently to describe products that contain the artificial sweetener Nutra-Sweet. Seems harmless enough on the surface, doesn't it? But I'll bet if I took a survey, I'd find that most consumers think that sugar free products are also calorie free, or, at the very least, low in calories. Unfortunately, this is not the case—a fact you'd be wise to remember the next time you start gobbling those benign little breath mints as a between meal snack. One roll of the sugar free variety can contribute almost 100 calories to your daily total!

Read... And Read Again!

For years now, I've been buying whole wheat bread instead of white bread. It is usually a richer source of fiber, vitamins and minerals than its paler counterpart. I also prefer the nutty flavor of most whole grain breads. But, I learned long ago to look specifically for the words *whole wheat* or *100% whole wheat*, and I will have to continue to take this precaution even with the new labeling requirements. Why? Because it's still perfectly legal for a baker to add, say, brown sugar to your old garden variety white flour in order to create a bread that is brown and *looks* like whole wheat. If you pick up a loaf that appears to be whole wheat but has only the word *wheat* on the label instead of *whole wheat*, you won't be purchasing what you thought you selected.

Healthy Is As Healthy Does

Healthy is what we all want to be—right? Food manufacturers know this, and so they wisely use this all-purpose description to decorate anything and everything that has any hope of landing on a supermarket shelf. And believe it or not, use of *healthy* is not covered under NLEA regulations! However, *healthy* will be defined under a separate proposal which is expected to be approved by May 1994. According to the definition used there, a food product that is low in fat and saturated fat, and has no more than 480 milligrams of sodium and 60 milligrams of cholesterol in one serving has earned the right to be called *healthy*. Until this restriction is in effect, my advice is to read the nutrition panel very carefully for any product that is described as *healthy*. Remember, it pays to be suspicious when it comes to health claims on food labels.

What You See Is Less Than What You Get

I know some of you found it nutritionally reassuring to read that interminable listing of vitamins on the old food label because it meant that every time you took a mouthful, you were being fortified. Take heart. Remember, our chief dietary problem today is one of excess—not lack. That's

48

why the new label puts the spotlight on fat, cholesterol, sodium and calories. It does not enumerate the levels of B vitamins, thiamin, riboflavin and niacin, because most Americans are getting sufficient amounts of these nutrients today. If a food is especially fortified with such nutrients or a manufacturer makes a specific claim that they are present, then they must be listed. Otherwise this level of detail is not required.

Many health experts agree with the new label's strong emphasis on macronutrients. Most are happy that Daily Value percentages for vitamins A and C, iron and calcium are included. But more than a few nutritionists are concerned that the importance of other vitamins and minerals is being downplayed. In another chapter, we will look at the roles that vitamins and minerals play in daily diets, so you can make certain you are getting what you need.

Folic Acid Faux Pas

Still other health experts feel that the FDA missed a chance for positive guidance by disallowing health claims linking folic acid to preventing neural tube defects like spina bifida and anencephaly in infants. What's confusing is that the FDA itself has recommended fortifying certain foods (e.g. flour) with folic acid to reduce the occurrence of neural tube defects. Apparently, further study is necessary in order to determine exactly what amounts of folic acid can be used safely.

High Fat vs. Low Fat

Yet another area of concern for conscientious health experts and nutritionists is the government's conclusion that fat should account for no more than 30% of a person's daily caloric intake. While it is true that the average American diet includes as much as 40% fat, and that 30% fat is certainly a step in the right direction, many who have made the study of healthful eating a career believe that our diets should include no more than 10 to 20% fat. Perhaps the wisest approach is to consider 30% fat a high fat diet and 10% fat a low fat diet, and then aim as low as possible. Once again, a chapter on weight loss will supply you with the information to hit your target diet.

Meat and Poultry Problems

For a while at least, you may encounter conflicting information when you consult labels on meat and poultry products and then turn to labels for non-meat products. For example, serving sizes may not follow the same guidelines. **Remember, the Nutrition Labeling and Education Act does not apply to meat and poultry products.** Labels for meat and poultry must adhere to regulations developed by the U.S. Department of Agriculture. However, the USDA has promised new labels that will "harmonize" with their non-meat counterparts.

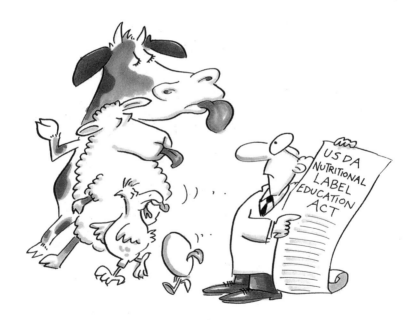

Smaller Is Not Necessarily Better

Take note that small food packages—less than 12 square inches—are exempt from providing nutritional information on their labels. So you can look for a listing of nutrients on that candy bar snack or the lunch-box-sized package of cookies, but don't be surprised if it is not there. Some manufacturers may, in good faith, include the basic **Amount Per Serving** figures, although they are not required to do so. What they *are* required to do is make certain their address and/or telephone number is somewhere on the packaging, so that you can write or call with any question you may have about the product.

Light Has More Than One Meaning

Here's an area that is bound to cause confusion, and, once again, it's the nutritionists who are crying *foul*. Under the NLEA regulations, *light* can mean fewer calories, less sodium or less fat. As if that were not enough work for one word, it can also be used to describe the texture or color of a food product, e.g. a ready-made frosting that is *light and fluffy*. So, consumer beware! When you see *light* on product packaging, check carefully to find out exactly what is *light*. Is it calories, fat, sodium or cholesterol? Or is it nothing more crucial that the product's ability to be whipped into frothy peaks? Clearly, the manufacturer has a responsibility to specifically state in what regard the product is *light*. If this fact is not made clear, I suggest shopping for another brand.

Free From Fat Fretting

Food products for children who are younger than two are in a special category also. Fat in general and saturated fat in particular may be substances most of us need to avoid, but the reality is that a very young child needs fat in order to grow and develop properly. The Food and Drug Administration did not want to give parents of this age group an indirect *and* mistaken message that infants and toddlers should join the rest of us on a restricted fat diet. Therefore, special regulations stipulate that labels for these products omit the figures for calories from fat and saturated fat.

Imagine! We all start out in this blissful state. For one brief, shining moment, we are free from fretting endlessly about fat, busily building up the strength and endurance we need to face a fat-free, or, at the very least, a fat-restricted future.

Meals Away From Home

Be sure to take into account the meals and snacks you consume that are not "home made." Manufacturers and preparers of food sold or served at the following sites are not required to provide nutritional information:

- Restaurants,
- Airplanes,
- Hospital cafeterias,
- Bakeries and delicatessens, and
- Stadium and sidewalk vendors.

For some of us—e.g., those gadabouts whose work requires travel—most food will be eaten "out." The sad fact is when you order your favorite pasta dish at a local trattoria, or grab a quick burrito during your lunch break, you won't be given a label with a nutritional accounting for your selection along with your check. In addition, chances are that neither the sauce on your pasta nor the cheese in your burrito are the low fat variety. If you eat out often, it would be wise to watch your diet carefully and make the low fat or fat free choice whenever you have that option. It's true that you will have to work a little harder than the average person in order to monitor your food intake, but your good health is worth the extra effort.

Read the Small Print!

I wish I could recommend a pill to protect you against the flood of health and disease-related claims that are bound to begin decorating the new food labels. Unfortunately, it's not that simple. All that I can offer you to combat the claims is information and some pretty homespun advice: *Proceed with caution!*

In 1906, the Food and Drug Administration imposed a ban prohibiting the use of health claims on food labels. At the time, this action was taken to curtail the deceptive practice of foods being sold as magical medicines. For example, in that less-than-scientific era, Grape Nuts cereal was actually marketed as a cure for, among other plights, appendicitis!

Well, 81 years have passed and—much to the delight of food manufacturers nationwide—the ban has been lifted. Health and disease-related claims may now adorn food labels once again. As you might expect, the reviews are mixed. The good news is that some foods *can* actually benefit the state of your health. And, you *do* need to know about these foods and their link to your well-being so that you can include them in your diet. The bad news? Well, there are some very thorny problems associated with this complex issue, and, to my knowledge, no one has really grappled with them yet.

We may not have solutions at this point, but we can profit from a clear understanding of the questions. Earlier this year, the University of California's *Berkeley Wellness Letter* did an excellent job of pinpointing some of the concerns that exist regarding health claims on food labels. Because I share their concerns, I'd like to pass them on to you:

• The first and most important question is one so basic that it almost escapes notice. Can a complex scientific explanation really be reduced to a single *accurate* phrase or statement? The obvious answer is *of course not*. Whatever the details, whatever the final slogan, it is not only unlikely, but also highly improbable that you are getting the whole story. If you accept and remember this fact and then approach your study of labels accordingly, you'll be a full step ahead of the claims game.

• Believe it or not, health claims intended for use on food labels do not have to undergo any kind of screening, nor are they obligated to obtain approval from the FDA before use. Manufacturers *are* forbidden to make "vague, unsubstantiated" assertions that a food actually cures a disease, but that's as tough as the regulations get. Forgive me if I seem cynical, but this is a fairly "vague" situation itself, one that will surely result in at least a few deceptive health claims finding their way to food labels, to supermarket shelves, and finally into your hands. How will the government deal with manufacturers who abuse this new right? How long will it take to get a product boasting a deceptive health claim out of circulation?

• Food manufacturers are cautioned to make certain that all health and disease-related claims are "science-based statements." What exactly does "science-based" mean? Who will judge whether a statement meets this criteria?

• Some foods contain one nutrient that is good for you and several others that are not. For example, it is true that butter contains vitamin A, and that the body needs vitamin A. But, butter also brings a lot of calories, fat and cholesterol to the meal—a high price to pay for a little vitamin A. Wouldn't you be better off eating a carrot or some apricots? That way, you'd get the vitamin A you need without the health risks associated with the excess calories, fat and cholesterol. The problem in this situation is that an unsuspecting and uninformed consumer may be taken in by a deceptive health claim on a package of butter, one that aggressively promotes the vitamin A content and conveniently ignores the other less beneficial nutrients.

• Finally, can one product or one nutrient actually improve the state of your health? The general consensus among health and nutrition experts seems to be *no*. Your health *can* benefit from good nutrition, they maintain, but only the cumulative total. The sum of right dietary choices over a period of years can really make a difference. That's fine. I can accept the fact that I have this lifelong responsibility to make healthful choices in the foods I eat. But, what about oat bran and its ability to reduce cholesterol levels? Or the fact that cranberry juice has been known to change the course of a bladder infection? In the end, I can only repeat: Read the fine print on every label, and read it carefully. Don't be gullible, but then again don't discount the nourishing, perhaps even healing properties of fresh, wholesome food.

Eat Right!

What to eat and how much to eat is information you will not find on the new food labels. There is, after all, only so much room on that panel! Putting the right foods together on a day to day basis in order to create a healthful diet is not something that should be left to chance. That's why I've included a separate section entitled *The Rest Is Up To You* in which I will tell you many things you'll need to know in order to accomplish this feat.

As I have pointed out, the new labels do have certain deficiencies, in and of themselves. In addition, nutrition labeling for most staples like fresh fruits and vegetables, fresh meat, poultry and fish is voluntary. I recently bought a beautiful bunch of fresh broccoli that sported its own abbreviated label. On a bright pink and white paper band that encircled the bunch, the grower or distributor (as the case may be) clearly listed the calories, protein, carbohydrate, fat, sodium, (all in grams) and potassium (in milligrams) contained in one stalk of fresh broccoli.

Now, I've been buying fresh broccoli and other fresh vegetables for years, but it was the first time I've ever seen an effort of this sort. I must admit that it warmed my heart. For one thing, I was impressed that the grower (or distributor) had seen fit to do something that was not required, to go "above and beyond the call of duty." The presence of that small label added to my growing conviction that we are, as a society, moving in what is clearly a more healthful direction with regard to what we eat on a daily basis. On a more personal level, I found it sweetly comforting to see that one stalk of fresh broccoli has only 50 calories and approximately .5 grams of fat. I considered my long time insistence that broccoli be our family's vegetable mainstay and felt suddenly wise and righteous. It was altogether a most positive and satisfying shopping experience!

Not all growers or manufacturers are going to provide nutritional information if they are exempt. The challenge for you lies in taking what information *is* provided and using it to create a diet that is both delicious and life enhancing. Keep reading. This book will give you the knowledge that is essential to this task.

THE REST IS UP TO YOU

It took years to make the new health-conscious labels a reality. But no matter how much relevant information is on the label, it will only benefit you if you take an active role in your health future. With the new labels, this has become easier to do.

Follow These Steps to Healthy Living!

Step One   Now that you know *how* to read the new food label, you're ready to...

Step Two   Actually *read* the labels and select the healthiest choices.

Start today. Read every frozen entree package, every cereal box, every can and bottle you pick up. Stock your refrigerator and cabinets with the most nutritious, low fat fare available in supermarkets today. Avoid the rest like the plague.

Great advice, you say—but how many people follow it all of the time? Can you really expect to make it all the way to the check-out line with an exemplary fat-free grocery cart every time you go shopping? Granted, nobody does all of the time, but you can certainly do it *some* of the time.

Consider using the 80/20 Rule of Good Nutrition.
If you make healthy choices 80% of the time,
you're allowed to indulge in sinful treats at least
20% of the time. Healthy choices all through your
work week means that you can savor that slice of
berry pie a-la-mode on the weekend. Make a deal
with me. Try the 80/20 Rule for at least two weeks,
and I predict you'll begin to notice something very
dramatic in your life. Because you haven't been
slathering your palette with non-nutritious fats and
sweets, you're actually going to be altering your
cravings for the stuff. It takes between three days
to one week for most people, but give this a chance.
You can alter your cravings for high fat, sugary
foods and improve your nutritional health 100%.

Because you're now a Certified Reader of Labels,
you can make the healthier choice between:

•　　La Choy Bi-Pack Chicken Teriyaki (2 fat
grams) and Lean Cuisine Baked Cheese Ravioli
(8 fat grams),

•　　General Foods Fruit and Fiber (2 fat grams)
and General Foods Corn Flake Toasties (0 fat
grams),

• Le Menu Salisbury Steak (9 fat grams) and Health Valley Vegetarian Chili with Beans (1 fat gram), and

• Green Giant Broccoli in Cheese Flavored Sauce (2 fat grams) and Green Giant Three Bean Salad (0 fat grams).

A difference of one or two fat grams between two choices may not sound like much, but over the course of a day, they tend to add up. In low fat living, every little fat gram counts.

Step Three   Now for your third and most challenging step—the real secret to improving your health in the long run: Commit to lifelong learning.

Fortify yourself with all the latest information regarding health promotion and diet. Studies have shown that those individuals who are most successful with long-term behavioral changes are the ones who actively seek out reinforcements for their modified stance. Consider the following information your first reinforcements supporting your new commitment.

Fact #1 The lower the fat content of the diet, the healthier it is in general.

Remember the struggle that ensued over how much fat the new food labels should advise people to eat in a day? Secretary Louis Sullivan had to do battle with powerful opponents who had ties to the meat and dairy industries. Eventually—and luckily for us—he won out with a label recommendation that Americans limit their fat intake to no more than 30% of their total calories.

But, the story doesn't end there. According to "Quaker Foresight," a consumer affairs newsletter published by the Quaker Oats Company, health and nutrition experts say dietary guidelines don't go far enough. *Consumer Reports* magazine asked 94 nutrition experts for advice on a theoretically ideal diet to promote health and reduce risk of disease. Most of the experts believe that fat consumption should be cut to less than 25% of daily calories, not the 30% or less currently recommended. Two-fifths of the experts think 20% would be better. Some experts offer very convincing evidence that 10% is the ultimate solution. Keep in mind, as mentioned earlier, that most Americans exist on diets that are rich with 36% to 40% of calories from fat.

Clearly, we all need to monitor the amount of fat we eat. If heart disease is already a health problem, reducing fat intake—especially saturated fat—offers the best hope of reversing it. If heart disease is not a problem, the right diet will help us avoid it.

But fat isn't the only nutrient that deserves our attention. Too much or too little of a variety of nutrients can have damaging effects over the long haul. Research shows that cancer, stroke, diabetes and atherosclerosis account for 68% of deaths annually. Government health officials estimate that between 50 and 80% of these early deaths might have been prevented through *proper diet*. Proper diet and the good health that comes with it is a result of making the right food choices. Before we can make the right choices, we must first of all know and understand what our choices are.

Fact #2 The healthiest diets include the "Golden Seven."

The truth is each day of our lives we need more than 50 nutrients from our food! Some nutrients—carbohydrates, protein and fat—serve as fuel by supplying calories. Others like fiber, vitamins, minerals and water play crucial roles in various body functions.

I don't know about you, but making certain I get the right amounts of 50 different nutrients seems like a pretty overwhelming task to me. I've always tried to keep in mind the latest advice from the U.S. Department of Agriculture's nutritionists when making choices. I look at the list as their Seven Golden Rules of Nutrition:

THE SEVEN GOLDEN RULES OF NUTRITION

1. Eat a Variety of Foods

2. Maintain Desirable Weight

3. Eat Adequate Starch and Fiber

4. Avoid Too Much Fat

5. Avoid Too Much Sugar

6. Avoid Too Much Sodium
7. If You Drink Alcohol, Do So in Moderation

Let's go over each of these briefly.

1.   Eat a Variety of Foods

Hundreds of gimmicky eating plans come and go, but researchers find that eating a variety of foods is the most nutritious means of achieving overall health and longevity. A diet deficient in nutrients increases the risk of developing certain diseases. This is the best reason to avoid fad diets, some of which can actually be dangerous.

A nutritious diet includes a wide variety of foods from each of the three caloric groups—carbohydrates, protein and fat—including sufficient vitamins, minerals, fiber and water. As we have seen, the FDA is currently recommending that your total daily calories be 30% fat, 15% protein and 55% complex carbohydrates. Personally, I agree with several nutritional and medical experts that you're better off with 20% fat, 15% protein and 65% complex carbohydrates. But if you're used to a diet of 45% fat, then curtailing it and loading up on the carbs—nutritious fruits, vegetables and grains—will be something you adjust to over time. And when you do, watch out—the health benefits will start pouring in. You better have a plan for all that extra energy!

2.   Maintain Desirable Weight

Good nutrition is important not only in keeping you healthy, strong and resistant to disease, but also in controlling your weight. Making certain you have several items from each food group each day is one way to begin to build a foundation of good nutrition. Your body needs this foundation to keep it running at its best and to feel satisfied—otherwise, your nutritional hunger may make you binge on non-nutritional, fattening snacks.

For a complete discussion on losing weight, read the chapter on weight loss.

3. Eat Foods With Adequate Starch and Fiber

Carbohydrates (starch) are the primary sources of energy for the body. There are of two kinds of carbohydrates: simple and complex. Carbohydrates include starch, vegetables, fruit and all forms of sugar. Complex carbohydrates (whole grains, pasta, legumes) serve as a long-acting fuel for the body. The American Dietetic Association and the National Institute of Health recommend that Americans increase their consumption of complex carbohydrates from the meager 25% that they've been eating to a level of 55% or higher. Carbohydrates provide only four calories per gram and are not as fattening as many people once believed. Carbohydrates are the exclusive fuel for brain function and are stored in the muscles as glycogen, which is used for short-term exercise. Carbohydrates are also "protein sparing," which means that when you consume adequate amounts of carbohydrates, your body is free to use dietary protein for tissue building and repair.

Carbohydrate sources are rich in nutrients, such as B vitamins and iron, as well as fiber. They also help promote a feeling of satiety or fullness. Sources of carbohydrates include breads, cereals, legumes, fruit, vegetables and milk. Complex carbohydrates consist of a chain of simple sugars and can be recognized as "starchy" rather than sweet. Sugars, such as glucose and sucrose, are carbohydrates but are nutrient-poor and for the most part contribute empty calories. These are called simple carbohydrates. The average American consumes far too much of this simple sugar —almost 124 pounds of sugar per year (much of it hidden in processed foods).

Fiber is obtained from whole grains, fruit and veg-etables. Fiber includes both the indigestible, crude type found in wheat bran and the water-soluble type found in beans and apples. It is important for promoting satiety, regulating bowel function, lowering cholesterol, regulating glucose absorption, and possibly reducing risk of certain bowel diseases. In general, the average American gets only 10 or 12 grams of fiber each day, much less than the 20 to 35 grams recommended by dietary experts.

If you don't take the time to get enough fiber in your diet, then by all means consider supplements. Fiber is simply too important to pass up due to a busy schedule or eating out all the time. And while you're taking fiber supplements, learn about the simple ways to adopt a healthy, low fat, high fiber diet. Include more legumes, oats, beans, oatmeal, apples, pears and strawberries in your diet—they are all excellent sources of fiber.

In the meantime, get fiber-regular. I've become a fan of psyllium supplements (made from a high fiber plant) and psyllium rich cereals and oat brans because of their abilities to serve as a gentle yet effective laxative agents, while also lowering blood cholesterol. These grains tend to attract water and form a gelatinous bulk, promoting regularity. Plus they interact with bile salts and other fat-related metabolic processes in the body to lower serum lipids. Most of the research on these two foods has been done at the University of Kentucky by Dr. James Anderson who found an 8.4% reduction in total serum cholesterol, along with a 12.9% reduction in low-density lipoproteins (LDLs—the chief culprits in atherosclerosis or coronary plaquing).

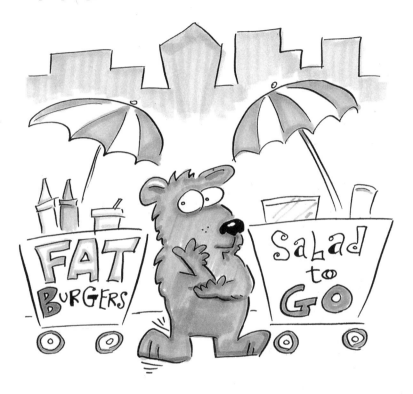

4. Avoid Too Much Fat

Fat is definitely the black sheep in today's nutritional pasture—but it really shouldn't be considered *bad*.

It's just that we eat far too many of the wrong kinds of fats. We're the ones out of control—not fat! It's a powerhouse of a nutrient; fat packs a whopping nine calories into every gram. Compare this to the mere four calories per gram stacked up by carbohydrates and protein. This condensed, calorie-rich nutrient is exactly the type of long-lasting, high endurance fuel sought by our nomadic, hunter-gatherer ancestors.

In times of long winters, food shortages or drought, those with the most fat on their bones were the ones that survived. That's why some scientists think that we might have selectively created a population with a high gene pool for obesity, or at least a tendency to store more body fat than we actually need today. After all, we're no longer running from saber-tooth tigers or trekking across tundras for an evening meal. So, it's important to choose our fats wisely.

Some types of fats are okay to consume, and others should be avoided. The three basic types of fats in foods are saturated, polyunsaturated and mono-unsaturated. It is important to limit your intake of **saturated** fats to less than 10% of your food intake a day or to no more than one third of your daily fat intake. In most cases, saturated fat comes into our diets in foods originating from animals. It is believed that these saturated fats affect the amount

AN OVERVIEW OF FOODS AND THEIR SATURATED FAT CONTENT

For your health and to maintain your optimal weight, select foods with low amounts of saturated fat.

Foods Essentially Free of Saturated Fat (Less Than 1 Gram)
Tortillas and flat breads
Grains
Vegetables
Fruits (except coconut and avocado)
Nonfat milk
Fat-free cheeses and yogurt
Beans
White fish (tuna in water)
Lean white turkey

Foods With Upper Limits of Saturated Fat
Fowl, dark meat
Most nuts
Cold cuts
Lean meats
Peanut butter
Large muffins
Bakery goods, refined sugar snacks
Processed snack foods (chips, crackers)
Corn and olive oil
Most salad dressings

Foods Loaded With Too Much Saturated Fat
Ice cream
Cream pies
Fast foods shakes
Fried chicken
Burgers with bacon and cheese
Steak
Taco salad with sour cream

of cholesterol that accumulates in our blood. Some foods from plant sources are also associated with increased blood cholesterol levels—including palm oil, palm kernel oil, and avocados. All are high in saturated fat.

Also limit foods high in **cholesterol**; this substance is found in animal fats, oils, and egg yolks. Elevated amounts of cholesterol in the bloodstream are associated with heart disease and stroke. Our own bodies produce as much cholesterol as we need. Excess cholesterol can deposit in arteries as plaque which increases the risk of heart disease.

Fats, carbohydrates and protein make up the caloric values of all foods. Proteins and carbohydrates each contain four calories per gram. Fat contains nine calories per gram—far denser.

CHECKLIST FOR CALORIES

- Carbohydrates   4 calories per gram
- Fat   9 calories per gram
- Protein   4 calories per gram
- Alcohol   7 calories per gram

Research shows that the proportions of each group that Americans eat is not particularly healthful.

The typical American diet has far too much fat and protein, and not enough complex carbohydrates. The simplest way to begin to consume healthier foods is to start eating twice as many fresh fruits, vegetables, whole grains and legumes as you cut back on fats and proteins.

5. Avoid Too Much Sugar

While most experts agree that sugar is not the "black hole" of nutrition it was once thought to be, everyone seems to benefit from reducing their consumption of refined sugars and foods high in sweeteners of all types. Instead of killing your appetite and filling up on sweets, which are usually high in calories and low in nutrients, try to substitute nutrient-rich foods. Sugar still deserves credit for being the body's quickest source of energy. However, too much of anything in one dose can stress your body's digestive and metabolic systems. For example, insulin production in the pancreas is significantly overtaxed from dealing with sudden increases in blood sugar levels. In addition, many report fewer mood swings, headaches and sugar cravings once they've elminated or reduced sweets. Whether sugar gives you the "highs" or the "blues," a little bit goes a long way. When you're craving something sweet, consider a ripe, juicy fruit or one of the new fruit-only frozen treats. Avoid products that load up on additional or artificial sweetners.

6. Avoid Too Much Sodium

To Salt or Not To Salt... Lately this issue has been very controversial. Some researchers think there has been a too far-reaching condemnation of the old salt shaker. Others disagree, pointing to the high amounts of sodium hidden in a variety of processed foods. I tend to agree with the low salt advocates. If your physician or nutritionist recommends you curtail your sodium intake, then by all means follow their advice to the letter.

The nutrient sodium earned a prominent place on the new food label because there are very real health risks associated with a high-salt diet. Whether you have high blood pressure or not, it pays to watch your sodium intake. The American Academy of Sciences tells us that we need anywhere from 1100 to 3300 milligrams of sodium each day. Contrast that range with the 4000 to 6000 milligrams that most Americans actually consume, and you have yet another example of our nationwide problem of dietary excess! Remembering these two facts helped me to cut down on my sodium intake. They can do the same for you.

WATCH THE SALT!
Recommended Amounts For Sodium

Actual	Recommended
4000 to 6000 milligrams a day*	1100 to 3300 milligrams a day*

- One teaspoon of salt contains 2000 milligrams of sodium — all you need for one day!

- Most processed foods already contain salt. If you add more, you're probably getting too much.

*Determined by the American Academy of Sciences as the range most Americans consume.

---

7. If You Drink Alcohol, Do So in Moderation

Watch out—alcohol is loaded with calories—7 calories per gram. For most people who drink alcohol regularly, they are always surprised how the pounds creep on. Sometimes it's not just the booze that adds weight, it's the snacking that goes along with social drinking. If you find yourself carrying extra weight, and you're sure that your diet is otherwise healthy (and your activity level is high), then consider cutting back on alcoholic beverages.

Then, of course, there's always the dependency factor. How often do you drink? Why do you drink? Do you enjoy an occasional glass of wine or a bottle of beer because you savor its taste, or do you retreat to it regularly to escape a tense situation? Honestly check out your drinking habits and take stock of a potentially risky behavior.

However, an occasional glass of premium wine can make an ordinary meal feel like a culinary feast. Enjoy alcoholic beverages in moderation.

Fact #3 A healthy diet not only prevents major diseases, it can help reverse a disease process.

At some of the top medical institutes in the U.S., the link between diet and disease is one crucial cornerstone of a revolutionary program that reverses heart disease. Participants of a yearlong study under the direction of the Preventive Medicine Institute in Sausalito, California actually unclogged their damaged coronary arteries without drugs or surgery! Although the study has ended, the original participants continue to come together for four hours one evening each week to review and reinforce the components of the program that made their recovery possible. The program included:

- Brisk walks,
- Yoga and meditation,
- Group support meetings,
- **An ultra-low-fat diet.**

Dr. Dean Ornish, president of the Preventive Medicine Institute and originator of its program, began dreaming of such a study while he was a student at Baylor College of Medicine Even though Ornish was lucky enough to observe state-of-the-art bypass surgeries performed by masters, he realized then that "bypasses bypassed the problem. They didn't cure heart disease." In other words, "If heart disease was an over-flowing sink, then bypass surgery was a better mop. I began wondering if there was a way to turn off the faucet."

John McDougall, M.D., another nutrition-friendly physician from Northern California, also found a way to "turn off the faucet." The celebrated McDougall Plan created daily "miracles" through a holistic approach. His regimen consisted of a low fat, vegetarian diet (which can be modified for those who cannot eliminate meat), relaxation, exercise and social support. In spite of the success of his diet, some consider these plans "impossible" for most Americans. I don't cotton much to the use of the word *impossible*, but I will go along with *difficult*. The diet contains a mere 10% of calories from fat—a real challenge for the average American who consumes close to 40% of calories from fat. Difficult, certainly. Impossible, not really.

Dr. Ornish claims that he has more than a thousand letters from people around the world who have read his book (*Dr. Dean Ornish's Program for Reversing Heart Disease*), adopted his program, and have watched their cholesterol drop and their chest pain lessen (and in some cases even disappear). Likewise, Dr. McDougall's book, *THE MCDOUGALL PLAN*, has found its way into the hearts of thousands—all with renewed hope for creating their own "turn-around" stories. Both of these physicians found that heart disease and other chronic illnesses were not only halted, but, in many cases, the fatty plaques were actually shrinking. The disease process had reversed!

Another person to consider if you're thinking about becoming a vegetarian is one of my favorite nutrition-friendly doctors—Michael Klaper, M.D. He wins friends and influences vegans everyday with his practical, down-to-earth message, cookbook and nutritional trouble-shooting advice. Read <u>Vegan Nutrition: Pure & Simple.</u> (ISBN 0-961428-7-7).

It's not only people with heart disease who can profit from the lessons learned by these conscientious physicians and their patients. We all can. A diet that is heart healthy should be everyone's top priority. And don't forget exercise! Incorporating regular aerobic exercise into your lifestyle is an essential component of maintaining your ideal weight and managing stress.

More Tips for Designing a Healthy Diet

Vitamin and Mineral Supplements—should you be taking them? If you're in good health and eat well-balanced meals from all food groups (cereals and grains, protein, dairy and fruits/vegetables), it's unlikely that you need to supplement your diet with vitamins and minerals. However, many nutritionists recommend a vitamin/mineral supplement if you tend to skip meals occasionally or not eat as well as you'd like. Megadoses are not necessary; in fact, they are dangerous. Large doses of vitamins A, B6 and D can be very toxic. The best prescription is to stay within the recommended norms.

I've really changed my thinking on vitamin and mineral supplements in the past few years. Like most health professionals, I pretty much followed the party line and said, "not necessary if you eat right." But then I started to record how people *really* eat today. How often do they take the time to prepare foods that are organically grown, ripe with nature's bounty, loaded with nutrients? How many of us are overburdened with hectic lifestyles that find us eating on the run, grabbing "something quick," skipping meals and, worse, eating junk?

I'm not making excuses. Nor am I advocating vitamins as insurance against the risks of a junk food diet. I'm just being a journalist and reporting what I see. Therefore, how much sense does it make anymore to keep telling people—eat right— when they're doing the best they can just picking up the right kids from child care! I don't want to be one more preachy voice coming from Unreal Land. When you're burning the candle at both ends, get yourself a high-stress nutritional insurance: take a daily supplement. No pill of course can guarantee health and well-being. And deficiencies aren't really what Americans are suffering with these days. But the simple act of stopping to take a vitamin/ mineral supplement will be your daily reminder to attend to your nutritional health. I hope.

Here are a few of the situations in which supplements make good sense. For example, if you're a men- struating women, an iron supplement helps replace the iron you lose when bleeding. Also, it's wise to take a calcium supplement, at least 1500 mg a day, to help maintain healthy bone structure and prevent osteoporosis. Women who are pregnant or who are breast-feeding need many more nutrients than they are able to consume, especially iron, folic acid, vitamin A and calcium. Their physicians and dietitians should give them detailed advice.

Exercisers Have Special Needs

Vitamins and minerals are organic compounds that are not made by the body but are required for growth, maintenance and repair of cells and tissues. For example, the B-complex vitamins help convert carbohydrate particles into energy molecules known as ATP. Vitamins C and E and the mineral iron are also important for sustaining good health in exercisers. As your exercise workload increases, adherence to a well-balanced diet grows increasingly important. Plus, there's good evidence to show that exercisers and anyone undergoing a high stress lifestyle could benefit from taking anti-oxidant supplements. Look for a generic brand of anti-oxidants and don't get talked up to "all-natural" or overly expensive brands.

Cut Back on Protein

Are you aware of the fact that most people in this

country overeat protein? Instead of having the recommended amount of 10% protein a day, the average American consumes a bloated, artery clogging 20 to 25%. Health experts are urging us to not only cut back on protein consumption but to also switch from a dependency on animal proteins (meat, poultry, dairy, fish) to vegetable proteins (grains, legumes and beans).

TARGETED AMOUNTS FOR PROTEIN
Per Day

Women	**RDA**
under age 24	46 grams
ages 25-70	46 to 50 grams

Men	
under age 24	less than 59 grams
age 25-70	63 grams

Americans are used to having large portions of meat on their plates. As a result, they consume between 65-105 grams on a daily basis—loading up their diet with too much cholesterol and saturated fat. Aim for around 50 grams of protein a day, and you'll meet the recommended requirement of 10% daily intake without any problem. Your 50 grams of protein might consist of 4 ounces of lean turkey on a sandwich at lunch and a 5 ounce serving of Filet of Sole at dinner (about the size of 1 1/2 decks of cards).

Note: You won't always see a "% Daily Value" across from the Protein category on the new nutrition label. Companies can volunteer that information but it is not required by the FDA.

Summary

Now you've got the basic tools to design a healthy diet for yourself and your family. Remember the 80/20 rule and enjoy a guilt-free splurge now and then. Squeeze the fat out of your diet and follow the Golden Seven. You'll be reducing your risk for chronic disease, while feeling lighter and more energetic everyday. The knowledge is in your hands; the commitment is up to you.

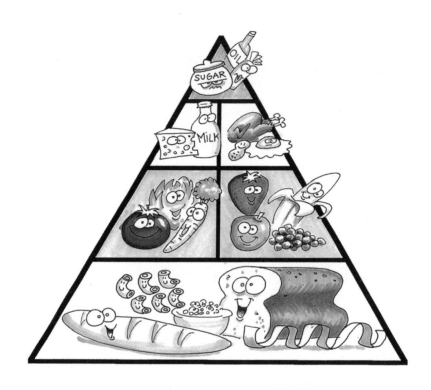

DISCOVER
THE NEW PYRAMID

Remember the "Basic Four" Food Groups? What grade school kid could ever forget it? Drummed in our brains from the first day we remembered our homework was the "Basic Four" philosophy. For over three decades the credo was that a healthy diet consisted of: Dairy, Meat, Breads and Grains, and Fruits and Vegetables.

The Basic Four Food Groups

1. Dairy
2. Meat
3. Breads and grains
4. Fruits and vegetables

This food planning system has been replaced by the Food Pyramid. (See opposite page and next page.)

For at least a decade the "Basic Four" has proven to be as outmoded a tool as the passive exercise table. In the light of new nutritional research, it was finally time to say good-bye to the Basic Four and hello to the new, improved, very up-to-date, highly desirable "Food Guide Pyramid."

Food Guide Pyramid

A Guide to Daily Food Choices

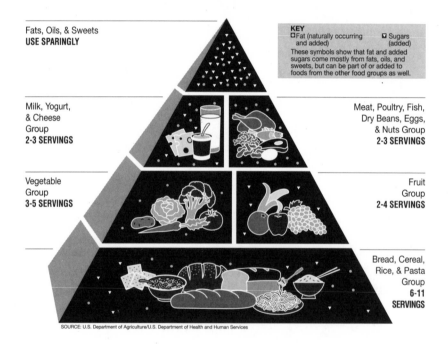

Fats, Oils, & Sweets
USE SPARINGLY

KEY
☐ Fat (naturally occurring and added)   ☑ Sugars (added)

These symbols show that fat and added sugars come mostly from fats, oils, and sweets, but can be part of or added to foods from the other food groups as well.

Milk, Yogurt, & Cheese Group
2-3 SERVINGS

Meat, Poultry, Fish, Dry Beans, Eggs, & Nuts Group
2-3 SERVINGS

Vegetable Group
3-5 SERVINGS

Fruit Group
2-4 SERVINGS

Bread, Cereal, Rice, & Pasta Group
6-11 SERVINGS

SOURCE: U.S. Department of Agriculture/U.S. Department of Health and Human Services

Courtesy: U.S. Department of Agriculture/U.S. Dept. of Health and Human Services

The Pyramid was issued in 1992 by the U.S. Department of Agriculture as a guide to good nutrition. Its purpose is to steer Americans away from their unhealthy high-fat diets to nutritionally balanced meals that contain more fiber and complex carbohydrates.

The Food Guide Pyramid takes the same information that makes up the food groups chart and rearranges it to make a point:

• Grains and cereals are the most important ingredients of a healthful diet.

• Foods are divided into five groups with suggested servings for each group.

• How much food you need each day depends upon your sex, age, physical condition and activity level.

• Most people need at least the minimum number of servings from each group daily.

SERVING SIZES FOR FOOD GROUPS
IN THE FOOD GUIDE PYRAMID

Food Group	Suggested Serving Sizes
Breads, Cereals, Rice and Pasta	6 to 11 servings 1 serving = 1 slice or 1/2 cup
Fruits	2 to 4 servings 1 serving = 1 piece fresh, 1/2 to 3/4 cup canned or juice
Vegetables	3 to 5 servings 1 serving = 1 cup raw leafy greens or 1/2 cup other vegetables
Meat, Poultry, Fish and Alternates (Eggs, Beans, Peas)	2 to 3 servings (total 5 to 7 ounces lean) A 3 ounce serving = 1 piece of meat about the size of a deck of cards.
Milk, Cheese and Yogurt	2 to 3 servings 1 serving = 1 cup or 1 1/2 ounces of cheese
Snacks, sweets, oils and fats	Minimal amounts if any

*Adapted from Dietary Guidelines for Americans. USDA, 1990.

Practice with the Healthy Eating Pyramid

If the government's Food Guide Pyramid still leaves you with unanswered questions when it's time to start cooking, there is a solution. The Center For Science in the Public Interest (CSPI) of Washington, D.C. has issued their own pyramid which is three dimensional. They claim their *Healthy Eating Pyramid* corrects the mistaken messages created by the USDA's 2-D triangle which makes no distinction between foods within a group. The government's food guide says, in effect, "As long as you have 2 to 3 servings a day from the milk, cheese and yogurt group, it doesn't really matter what you eat. A frozen yogurt sundae or a glass of non-fat milk have equal status.

CSPI's Healthy Eating Pyramid, on the other hand, separates the healthiest foods from the unhealthiest ones based on their content of fat, saturated fat, cholesterol, sugar and salt. Specific foods are placed either on the *Anytime*, *Sometimes*, or *Seldom* sides of this nutrition aid.

The pyramid defines its categories this way:

• *Anytime* - Foods in this elite group should be the backbone of your diet. Examples are pasta, whole-grain bread, fish and most vegetables and beans. Most are low in fat (oily fish is the exception) and saturated fat and have no serious flaws.

91

• *Sometimes* - Foods that land on this side of the pyramid are neither your best nor your worst choices. Only small portions and no more than two or three servings a day of foods like white bread, fig bars, turkey bologna, and potato salad are recommended.

• *Seldom* - Your worst fears are confirmed! How does the chart rate that quarter-pound cheese-burger, your favorite chili, and those chocolate sand-wich cookies you've been eating since childhood? Yes, they're all here on the only *occasionally* or *rarely* side, and even then only small portions are suggested.

The Healthy Eating Pyramid gives you a lot of information about healthy eating in simple and direct language that even a child can understand. For example, instead of all chicken being in one group, you'll find a skinless chicken breast on the *Anytime* side of the pyramid; a skinless, but fattier chicken thigh on the yellow *Sometimes* side; and a thigh with skin on the red *Seldom* side. After all, not all chicken parts are equal.

The CSPI and the USDA do agree on one funda-mental point: Americans need to eat more grains, vegetables and fruit but fewer dairy products and less meat.

The *Healthy Eating Pyramid* ranks foods first on their fat content. Then, foods that are high in salt, sugar or cholesterol are moved down one category. The end result is a nutritional aid that makes your health its top—and only—priority. Worry-free meal planning can be yours with a quick glance at the *Anytime* side of the pyramid.

The CSPI has made their ingenious *Healthy Eating Pyramid* available to help you with meal planning. You can order a sturdy paper copy from the non-profit, health-advocacy organization by sending $5 to CSPI Pyramid, Suite 300, 1875 Connecticut Ave. NW, Washington, DC 20009-5728. A more durable plastic version is available for $15. You can also order either CSPI Pyramid by phone. Call CSPI at (202) 332-9110.

Here's to Healthy Eating

A basic understanding of the new food label and CSPI's *Healthy Eating Pyramid* will help you translate general nutrition advice like "less fat" and "more fiber" into healthy meals.

Once you do, you'll be able to enjoy the unique experience of *happily* eating healthy food. For those of you doubting Thomases who think this phenom-enon is just not possible, consider the culinary surprise I found at my local shopping mall the other day. Determined to find a low-fat alternative to the double chocolate chip cookie that is my traditional reward for a day spent shopping, I took a quick inventory of the fanciful food concessions. A slice of pizza? No, not quite. French fries and a coke? I think not! But wait, what's that sign on the frozen yogurt counter? A *Slimdae*? "Is that anything like a sundae?" I asked the childlike clerk behind the cash register. "Not really," she responded brightly. "With a Slimdae, you get six ounces of non-fat yogurt topped with a 99% fat-free hot fudge sauce—all for only 130 calories! Like to try one?" Now I ask you, what would you have said? Well, I decided to try the *Slimdae* and am happy to report I did not feel disappointed or deprived. In fact, I felt every bit as rewarded as I had in the past with the fat-filled "real thing."

So, take heart. If scientists and nutritionists can work together to accomplish such feats with food, we can obviously look forward to a future that is both nutritious *and* delicious!

GUIDELINES FROM THE AMERICAN HEART ASSOCIATION

30% or less calories from FAT
10% or less calories from SATURATED FAT
150 mg or less CHOLESTROL
1100 mg or less SODIUM

WEIGHT LOSS &
THE FOOD LABEL
A LOVE STORY

Are you sick and tired of all of those ridiculous gimmicks and quick weight loss promises shouted by the $40 billion diet industry? I am. Ignore them. I'm going to give you one rule of thumb that works for 99% of the people 99% of the time.

**To Lose Weight, Eat Less Fat
and Increase Your Activity.**

That's all there is to it. This really isn't brain surgery, folks. Don't fall for diet plans that insist on their own prepackaged frozen meals. Disappointed dieters rarely learn to choose wisely, select with confidence, and prepare meals according to your own hard-earned low fat wisdom. Which leads me to the second point:

**To Eat Less Fat, Buy Less Fat.
READ THE LABEL.**

Pay special attention to the top portion of the label that gives you the facts about calories, calories from fat, total fat content and saturated fat content.

NUTRITION FACTS

Serving Size 2 ounces
Servings Per Container 6

Amount Per Serving
Calories 220   Calories from Fat 27

	% Daily Value
Total Fat 3 g	5%
Saturated Fat 0.5 g	2%

---

1. Does this food have more calories than you want?
2. What's the percentage of its calories that are derived from fat?
3. How much saturated fat does it contain?

FORMULA
TO DETERMINE THE
PERCENTAGE OF
FAT CALORIES

Total Calories Divided	$\underline{220}$
by Calories from Fat	27

= 8 % Fat Calories

96

For overall calorie intake, you really shouldn't dip below 1200 to 1500 calories per day on any weight loss program without your physician's supervision. Drastic calorie-reducing diets tend to slow metabolic processes to the point in which your body goes into a survival mechanism, and begins to store fat like crazy. Then, just when you thought it was safe to eat normal amounts again, all the pounds return and then some.

You're better off eating a healthy amount of calories and concentrating on reducing your fat intake instead. Here's how! Become a quick division expert, and get used to dividing the number of Total Calories (for example, 220) by the number of Total Calories from Fat (let's say 27) to get the percentage of that item which is made up of Fat Calories (8%). This information will help you select low fat items.

You can also work with the % Daily Value figures presented on the new label to reduce your fat intake. Keep your average % daily value for fat to 5% or less, as we usually eat about 20 items throughout the day.

You should also pay close attention to the bottom of the label. It serves as a reminder for you to count your fat grams if you are so inclined. A 2000 calorie diet is not easy to lose weight on unless you're doing at least 1-2 hours of exercise per day. It would be more advantageous to think about taking in 60 grams or less of total fat, and 20 grams or less of saturated fat.

MORE ON FAT
ON THE NEW LABEL

Calories	2000	2500
Total Fat Less Than	65g	80g
Sat. Fat Less Than	20g	25g
Cholesterol Less than	300mg	300mg
Sodium Less Than	2400mg	2400mg
Total Carbohydrate	300g	375g
Dietary Fiber	25g	30g

Calories per gram:

Fat 9   •   Carbohydrate 4 •   Protein 4

You should also be doing your best to increase your intake of fresh fruits, vegetables and whole grains, and decrease the empty calories: sugary snacks, high fat chips, dips, creamy salad dressings, ice cream, cookies, donuts and high fat dairy products. As I mentioned earlier, fats are a calorie-dense food. One gram of fat contains nine calories. Therefore, fat-laden meals can add a tremendous amount of calories to your daily intake even though it may appear you are eating normal quantities of food. A hamburger fried in grease, with oil-drenched french fries, and a saturated-fat milkshake together contain four times the calories of a meal consisting of fresh salad, applesauce, steamed vegetables, broiled fish and iced tea with sugar.

You can easily limit your fat calories to less than 30% by following this formula: Calorie intake x 0.3 / 9 = your maximum grams of fat per day. For example: 2000 cal. x 0.3 = 600 / 9 = 67 grams of fat per day. Another interesting tidbit: Calculating half of your ideal weight (120 / 2 = 60) can help you figure out your total daily caloric need. Just multiply the total by three (60 x 3 = 180) and add a zero (1800 calories per day).

HOW TO FIGURE YOUR HEALTHY LOW FAT INTAKE

Limit your fat calories to less than 30%
by following this formula:

Calorie intake x 0.3 / 9 = Your maximum grams
of fat per day

Examples:

2000 cal. x 0.3 = 600 /9 = 67 grams of fat per day

1600 cal. x 0.3 = 480 / 9 = 54 grams of fat per day

How Do You Know
Your Desirable Weight?

The best advice these days is to forget about your
weight, and get your body fat measured instead.
You can do this at any health club or sports clinic.
You could also ask physician about it. The conven-
tional height and weight tables show desirable
ranges for most adults, but they really don't address
something that health professionals have known for
over two decades: it's your body composition that
matters—not your weight. What needs to be measured is how much body fat do you have compared
to lean mass such as bones and muscles.

If your body fat measurements are in an average
range, and you still think you need to lose weight,
then consider what other forces may be at play in
your life. Constant cultural and media pressures on
women and men to be thin has led professionals to
rethink our approach to weight counseling. We're
finding out that three out of five women are always
on diets—just because they *think* they're fat. Studies
have shown that 70% of women are dissatisfied
with their weight and 80% diet for the sake of
appearance rather than health. The Centers for
Disease Control in Atlanta found that almost two-
thirds of chronic dieters were not overweight when
they began dieting.

The obsession with thinness has affected young people so adversely that eating disorders begin as early as 6 to 8 years of age in girls.

So, if you're well within a healthy range, then work on your body image instead, stop the negative self-talk and give your body a break. I suggest Dr. Ellen McGrath's *When Feeling Bad Is Good* (published by Henry Holt)—and I humbly speak from experience.

When Are You Overfat?

According to Dr. Frank Katch who directs the Department of Exercise Science at the University of Massachusetts, the following numbers are the upper limits of normal levels of body fat: for men, over 20%; and for women, above 30%.

Dr. Katch and Dr. William McArdle are two of the nation's leading experts in human nutrition and body composition. Their recent writings all point to body distribution as an indicator for certain health hazards (diabetes, heart disease, high blood pressure, and high blood lipids).

One way of evaluating your body distribution is to grab a tape measure and determine your **waist-to-hip-ratio.** This is always good for a self-honesty test if nothing else. And to measure abdominal obesity, divide the waist measurement (at the navel) by the hip (over the widest part of your butt). Ideally, the waist should not be larger than the hips. Results above 0.95 for men and 0.80 for women are associated with greater risk, according to the *Obesity & Health Journal.*

By far the most inaccurate measurement of your fatness is to stand naked in front of the mirror and evaluate your physique—even though that recommendation is as old as "diet" drinks. We are our own worst critics, unrelentingly judgmental and unforgivingly harsh. Stick with a professional's body fat measurements. You may be pleasantly surprised. And if you're not...read on.

How Do You Lose Weight?

Well, first and foremost, if you've been a chronic dieter, don't ever diet again. Dieting has become such a serious concern for women and men that they run greater risks for heart disease and total deaths due to weight cycling or yo-yo dieting, accord-ing to an analysis of 32 years of data from the famous Framingham study. What you need is a healthful way of eating, a routine of consistent, moderate exercise and a new relationship to food!

This is all garnered through support groups, counseling from qualified nutritionists and well-informed, nutrition-friendly physicians, and getting a good self-education—just as you're doing now.

Fad diets, low calorie liquid meals, pre-packaged frozen diet meals all have a poor record for long-term success. *They* fail *you* in the long run, even though you feel like a failure. So-called weight loss programs that fail to teach you new and better habits of eating and exercise makes as much sense as teaching pigs to whistle. Don't fall for them.

Become Friends with Exercise

No weight loss program is worth its weight that doesn't recommend daily exercise. In the long run, increasing your calorie output through consistent, sweat-producing exercise is one of the most significant means of weight management. But don't exercise so you can overeat later. Exercise in and of itself is a tough way to lose a lot of weight. Exercise combined with a sensible low fat eating plan is the optimal choice. And it doesn't end there. Five years ago health professionals used to recommend aerobics for weight loss because aerobic exercise is known to burn fat. But today, many professionals are also recommending strength training or muscular endurance classes for weight loss. As you increase the size and strength of your lean muscles, your body becomes more efficient at fat-burning in general. Today there are many recruits, including women, to a combination workout—aerobics plus muscle conditioning. They swear that this combined workout gets rid of fat in places that the aerobics-alone routine never touched.

Aside from slimming down and losing fat, consistent enjoyable exercise has a remarkable impact on your overall health and psycho-emotional spirits. Make sure your exercise plan includes the FIT principle—which looks at Frequency, Intensity and Time. Under the FIT principle, you'll target a frequency of 4 to 5 times a week. Your intensity of exercise, when working at a training range, should usually be about 60 to 85% of your maximal heart rate. Start at timed sessions of 20 minutes and work up to 60. You'll want to alternate 3 days of aerobics (cycling, treadmill, walking, jogging and running) with at least 2 days a week of strength training (body shaping, resistance machines, conditioning classes and free weights.)

Alternate 3 days a week of aerobics (cycling, treadmill, walking, jogging and running) with at least 2 days a week of strength training (body shaping, resistance machines, conditioning classes and free weights).

THE FIT PRINCIPLE
FOR EXERCISE

F: Frequency — 4-5 times per week

I: Intensity — Work at your training range, usually about 60-85% of your maximal heart rate

T: Time — Start with 20 minutes then aim for 60 minutes at a session

Summary

There really are no short cuts to weight management. You've got to consider adopting a long-term health life-style approach. Deprivation does not work. It sets you up for problems in the long run, leading to more frustration and anger. Become aware of why you eat; there are all sorts of psychological reasons to eat. Once you've uncovered those, realize that you can't always get the satisfaction you want from food. But when you have a physiological hunger, relax and enjoy your food.

As long as you follow the Principles for Successful Weight Loss listed in the next chart, you will be correcting your weight naturally. And best of all, you'll be achieving glowing health.

STRATEGIES FOR SUCCESSFUL WEIGHT LOSS

- Eat a variety of foods that are low in calories and high in nutrients.

- Read labels for fat, saturated fat, cholesterol and total calories. Choose the lowest amounts you can find. Keep total fat intake less than 30% and saturated fat less than 10%.

- Don't try to lose weight rapidly—it will rebound on you. Aim for a weight loss of 1/2 to 2 lbs per week.

- Practice new habits to control overeating: eat slowly, take smaller portions, and avoid seconds.

- Eat less fatty foods. Avoid high fat snacks, cookies and bakery goods.

- Eat less sugar and sweets.

- Find nonfat substitutes for butter, ice cream, oils, salad dressings, cheese and yogurt.

- Drink less alcoholic beverages. (They're loaded with empty calories!)

- Exercise, exercise, exercise.

HEALTH CONCERNS AND THE NEW LABEL

Now that more people are growing health-conscious, they're learning how to better manage many illnesses and chronic conditions that they used to feel powerless about and handle by turning them over to the medical profession with complete resignation. But with the new nutrition label, there is an opportunity to become your own health champion, taking more control and looking at nutritious foods as central players in the healing process. Reading labels can improve your health and save your life in any number of ways!

If you have any one or more of the following health conditions, be sure to pay special attention to the area(s) listed below. In fact, get accustomed to initially scanning certain sections of the label automatically.

If you have...   Check the Label for...

Cancer risk   **Fat and Saturated Fat**
                           Unsaturated Fat (if listed)

Diets high in fat are associated with certain cancers in vast population studies, although the direct causal evidence is not all there yet. But in the meantime, many health experts consider it prudent for anyone at risk for cancer to cut back on fat intake. This includes both saturated and poly-unsaturated fats. For all those interested in lowering their cancer risk, as well as those who are undergoing cancer treatment, make friends with the cruciferous vegetables. These include cauliflower, Brussels sprouts, kale and broccoli. Researchers are proving they may be protective against certain cancers. You won't find labels on any of these vegetables, other than an educational sign promoting health benefits posted by a nutrition-friendly store. You also want to load up on anti-oxidants, found abundantly in fruits, vegetables and grains. These help the body neutralize any damage done by free radicals, incomplete byproducts of metabolism that destroy cells and genetic material. Also, avoid char-broiled foods and cut back on alcohol.

If you have...	Check the Label for...
Colon Cancer	**Dietary Fiber**
Constipation	
Diverticulosis	
Intestinal Disorders	

Fiber is the only nutrient that the rest of the "undeveloped" world gets enough of, and that Americans can't seem to find in their diets. All the diseases linked with a low intake of fiber in the Western nations are nonexistent in the parts of the world with a high-fiber intake, especially colon cancer. Maintaining adequate amounts of fiber in the daily diet can help many different kinds of gastrointestinal disorders, but be sure to check with your physician first. Most Americans have a meager fiber intake of less than 15 mg. Increase your fiber intake slowly, working up to 35 mg a day. Many ailments are also aggravated by high fat intakes. Limit your fat calories to 30% of your daily caloric intake, or less if you can.

If you have...	Check the Label for...
Heart Disease	**Fat and Saturated Fat**
Family History	**Cholesterol**
of Heart Disease	**Sodium**

If you have heart disease, you should select foods with low amounts in these three categories. If you don't know why, see your physician or a registered dietitian. If you have a family history of heart disease, then it's wise to alter your diet to a low-fat one immediately. The link between dietary intake of saturated fats, cholesterol and triglyceride (a common fat found in foods) as a contributing factor in developing high cholesterol levels, and, in turn, cardiovascular disease is strong. There are some exciting studies of heart disease being halted and even reversed through a vegetarian diet providing no more than 10% of its calories from fat. Heart patients with congestive heart failure also need to check the sodium content of foods, aiming as low as possible.

If you have...	Check the Label for...
High Cholesterol	**Fat and Saturated Fat Cholesterol**

The front of the package may be blasting "low fat, no cholesterol!" but you've got to read the small print in the nutrition label. That's the only place you can trust to deliver the information you need. This is where you want to read nothing but zeroes for Fat, Saturated Fat and Cholesterol. Many food packages will boast that they're "cholesterol free," but shouldn't really need to tell consumers this information. For example, ketchup doesn't need animal products and therefore should never have cholesterol. Buying a product simply because it claims no cholesterol is falling for slick advertising. Check the fat and saturated fat categories as well since they raise cholesterol levels significantly.

If you have...   Check the Label for...

Hypertension   **Sodium**

If high blood pressure is your concern, learn to track the sodium content on everything you buy. **The word "unsalted" on the front of the label does not mean that the product doesn't contain sodium. Always check the label.** Examples of high sodium food are frozen pizza slices with 1000 mg per slice. Medium sodium content would be margarine with 120 mg per tsp. A low sodium example is any fruit with 2-5 mg per entire piece. Beware of soft drinks—they don't taste salty but many are loaded with sodium. A large can of soup can supply the entire 2400 mg for the day! One frozen dinner can also contain as much as 80% of the day's sodium intake. The FDA has recommended 2400 mg per day as the maximum amount for healthy individuals. Doctors often recommend much less than that (under 2000 or 1500) for people who need to cut back.

If you have...   Check the Label for...

Osteoporosis   **Fat and Saturated Fat**
                        Cholesterol
                        Calcium (may not be listed)

Osteoporosis is not attributable to one thing such as

a lack of calcium. It's the result of an entire range of factors, including an inevitable thinning of bones with aging. To prevent the ravages of osteoporosis, don't smoke cigarettes, take plenty of calcium, limit alcoholic drinks, exercise daily, and consider hormone replacement therapy. As far as the Nutrition Label is concerned, you need to be aware of these points: Plentiful sources of calcium are usually the products which are also high in fat—dairy (milk, yogurt, cheese) and beef. Look for the nonfat or low-fat versions of these products. Often the nondairy substitutes made to look and taste like dairy products contain too many artificial ingredients. Most of your best foods won't have labels. Top choices among vegetables are beet greens, Swiss chard, collars, spinach, turnip greens, broccoli and kale. Other good sources of calcium: salmon, sardines, almonds, figs, soybeans and tofu. One of the lowest sources is cottage cheese! Calcium recommendations are 800 mg a day for adults, 1200 mg a day for children, young adults and women who are pregnant or lactating. And recently a new recommendation has emerged for post-menopausal women of 1200 to 1500 mg of calcium a day. Here is where supplements may be necessary since most people have an intake of 600 mg of calcium per day.

<u>If you have...</u>   <u>Check the Label for...</u>

Diabetes   **Carbohydrates**
Hypoglycemia   **Sugar**
Sugar Sensitivity

High levels of blood sugar can cause everything
from fatigue, drowsiness and light-headedness to
hyperactivity, anxiety and coma in people who have
difficulty converting and storing simple sugars or
glucose. All carbohydrates whether they are complex ones found in whole grain breads or the simple
ones such as fructose (found in fruit) and lactose
(found in milk) break down to form simple glucose
in the body. There really is no such thing as a bad
sugar or a good sugar. The calories from a slice of
bread and the calories from Kool-Aid wind up
providing energy through the same pathway. The
problem with sweet-tasting food is that it is usually
non-nutritious because it is missing vitamins,
minerals, fiber and other elements. If you are trying
to curtail your intake of sugar, then you need to
read both carbohydrates and sugar content.

Diabetics are also advised to keep their saturated fat
intake to a minimum. Higher intake of low-fat
proteins and foods high in water-soluble fiber are
often recommended to smooth out the highs and
lows of erratic blood sugar levels.

TEST YOUR LABEL AWARENESS

Well, now you're a Certified Label Reader, and there's no stopping you. Make a vow to read every label on everything you consider buying for the rest of your life! Teach your friends and family to read labels. Teach your co-workers to read labels. Show that beloved Yorkie stuffed in your purse the label on the dog food you're considering for him. Become a fanatic about labels. Turn into a living, label fable. Write a comedy routine about the nonsense you find between the hype on the front and the truth in the small print. Impress your friends with your nutritional laser-like label wit.

In summary, you know what food labels can do for you, and the rest is up to you. They supply you with the information on ingredients, serving size, weight and other specifics. What else? They have the potential of helping you discern whether the product's advertising is false or misleading. Advertising, as you know, is meant to capture your attention and highlight certain advantages. And lately, advertisers have been working over-time to communicate a message that lets you believe the food manufacturer has your healthiest interests in

115

mind. Every manufacturer of air-puffed chips and instant liquid meals with hidden hydrogenated oil would have you believe that their latest concoction is "naturally nutritious." That kind of claim is always going to be around. When in doubt, check the label.

For example, imagine a baby food ad that shows a picture of a baby sitting in a field with pesticide-spraying planes dousing her from overhead, and says, "It's important to buy our baby food because her safety depends on it. " The advertisement contains an implied safety or reliability claim. (Buy any other type of baby food, and you may be stuffing pesticides into your little darling.) The Federal Trade Commission initiates law enforcement action against claims that are considered misleading, especially when there is no supporting evidence to back them up. But they can't protect you at every turn. The FTC has a long list of claims, a limited amount of researchers and prosecutors, and consumers are usually at the mercy of untruthful claims for quite a while before they are off the shelf or disappear from the airwaves.

THE NEW LABEL
Nutrition Facts

NUTRITION FACTS

Serving Size 2 ounces	
Servings Per Container 6	

Amount Per Serving	
Calories 220	Calories from Fat 27

	% Daily Value *
Total Fat 3 g	5%
Saturated Fat 0.5 g	2%
Cholesterol 54 mg	20%
Sodium 28 mg	1.2%
Total Carbohydrate 40 g	13%
Dietary Fiber 0 g	-
Sugars 1 g	-
Protein 8 g	-

* Percent Daily values are based on a 2000 calorie diet. Your daily values may be higher or lower depending on your calorie needs:

		Calories	2000	2500
Total Fat	Less than		65 g	80 g
Sat Fat	Less than		20 g	25 g
Cholesterol	Less than		300 mg	300 mg
Sodium	Less than		2400 mg	2400 mg
Total Carbohydrate			300 g	375 g
Dietary Fiber			25 g	30 g

Calories per gram:

Fat 9 • Carbohydrate 4 • Protein 4

LABEL QUIZ

So what have you learned so far? Here's a chance to put your label-sleuthing skills to work. Go to work, Certified Label Reader. Discover the real meaning of food.

1. What's the healthier snack?

    Tortilla chips
    Microwave popcorn
    Pretzels
    Graham crackers

2. You run across something in the refrigerated section of your supermarket with a label that screams, "Reduced fat!" What a find! This means the food has 3 grams of fat or less per serving.

    True _____   False _____

3. You feel like having rice tonight. You know you've only got white rice at home, and you understand that brown rice is healthier. What's the better choice of these two?

    a. Boil the white rice.
    b. Prepare a box of Savory Classics from Rice-a-Roni.

4. Easy and convenient—that's what the overworked consumer is seeking Monday through Friday. What better way to fix an easy meal than to pour a bottle of Ragu sauce over chicken...hence, Ragu's Chicken Tonight. Pick up the bottle of Salsa Chicken, and you read "0 grams of fat." Sounds great. Ahh...but what's this? Ragu's Country French Chicken. Sounds even better. Throw that one in the basket. What's wrong with this picture.

    _____ (an essay question)

5. Since you've been told to avoid cholesterol, you make sure you buy cholesterol-free products. Otherwise, you don't worry about the fat content of foods. You are:

    a. A savvy shopper. Continue to steer clear of animal fats.
    b. A poor misguided fool. Reduce both fat and cholesterol!

6. You're interested in losing weight. The low-fat granola cereal sounds better than your old staple, Cheerios. And after reading the label, you discover that the two cereals are almost equal in calories and fat content. You buy the granola. Was it a leaner, healthier choice?

    a. Yes
    b. No

ANSWERS

1.   A tough question because there's several lousy choices. Here's a case for the advanced label detective. Tortilla chips come in a few varieties; be sure to read the nutrition facts carefully. The new baked chips contain no oils but generally taste like cardboard. If you can stand them, they're a fat-free snack. Microwave popcorn is dripping with fats, and the worst kind of saturated or hydrogenated fats at that. Get an air popper and make your own popcorn instead. Pretzels without salt are usually a healthy snack. The ones with salt granules the size of your fist are way over the top for sodium limits. Don't despair. There are some healthy new varieties of graham crackers with a zero fat content.

2.   False. Sorry, this may not be the low fat treasure you thought it was. All "reduced fat" means is that the food has been processed to reduce its fat content by 25% or more from what it previously contained. The worst scenario is that it may contain 75% fat!

3.   In terms of whole grain nutrition, it's a toss up. You're not getting whole grains in either package. The Savory Classics features long grain rice, not the same as a whole grain. In terms of fat content, you're better off with the white rice at home.

Preparing the fancy flavored box rice as directed will give you 4 grams of fat per serving. In this case, a serving is estimated to be only 1/2 cup. Not many people stop at a half-cup of rice. You could easily be ingesting 8-12 grams of fat in a dish that traditionally is fat free!

4.   Not all jars of simmer-and-serve are created equal. The white sauces are usually heavier in fat content. In this case, Country French Chicken not only has 12 grams of fat compared to Chicken Salsa's 0 grams, but it also has 5 milligrams of cholesterol compared to 0 in the red sauce. The lesson here: Be sure to read the label on the exact package you're buying, not just its sister flavor.

5.   b. If you are told by your doctor to curtail your cholesterol intake, you're probably doing so to lower your risk of heart attack and stroke. You may have an excessive dietary intake of cholesterol, but chances are you are coping with an inherited predisposition to high serum levels of cholesterol. Perhaps your liver simply manufactures an excess amount. Since the liver's production is significantly influenced by the your intake of dietary fat, you can take an important measure to safeguard your health by lowering your intake of all fats: vegetables oils and fats (which do not contain cholesterol) and animal fats (the cholesterol culprits).

6.   b. No, sorry. You were right to check the label for calorie and fat content. But when it comes to cereal, don't stop there! The recommended serving size for these cereals is one ounce by weight. Pour an ounce of feather-light, little Cheerios in your bowl, and you get a full 1-1/4 cup—a normal serving for most of us. But take those heavy-weight granola cereals and measure one ounce. You're left with a meager 1/3 cup! And nobody stops there. Fill your bowl the same way with the granola cereal, and suddenly you've pigged out on 3 to 4 times the calories and fat content found in your old pal, Cheerios.

A Final Pep Talk -
Here Whenever You Need It

Changing habits is never easy. We need all the help we can get at times. Let this page serve as an affirmation for your commitment to healthier living. Read it whenever you need a motivational boost.

I'm in Charge.

I know how to make choices according to the helpful information on the new food label.

I use it wisely to help me maintain good health and prevent disease.

I educate myself about the food I eat and the environment I live in—two factors that strongly affect my health.

And I am the one who knows what really keeps me healthy. Not food alone—my health also depends upon mental hardiness, emotional resilience and spiritual strength.

I embrace a holistic approach which allows me to attain levels of optimal health many only dream about.

Stay well!

RESOURCES

To help you make the best use of the information you now know how to find on the new labels, I've compiled a list of resources for information on labeling, nutrition and healthy living. Browse through, and you'll find the sources for a number of tools—such as the CSPI Healthy Eating Pyramid (mentioned earlier in this book). A suggested reading list of books and periodicals is also provided as well as some quick reference charts.

BOOKS

Good Food Today, Great Kids Tomorrow: A Pediatrician's Guide to 50 Things You Can Do For Happy, Healthy Children by Jay Gordon, M.D. and Antonia Boyle. Available from Michael Wiese Productions, 4354 Laurel Canyon Blvd., #234, Studio City, CA 91604 (818) 379-8799.

BRAND NAME GUIDES

For the most comprehensive list of the fat content in commercially processed foods:

The Fat Counter by Annette Natow and Jo-Ann Heslin
  Pocket Books (paperback)
  Over 10,000 entries including packaged and frozen foods, fast foods from major chains, and prepared mixes and snacks.

Nutrition Coordinating Center
Brand Names booklet
University of Minnesota
2221 University Ave., SE, Suite 310
Minneapolis, MN 55414-3076
(612) 627-4862

DINING OUT

Heart Smart Restaurants International offers low fat, low cholesterol and low sodium choices. Find out the restaurants that qualify near you. Call toll-free (800) SMART-19.

HEALTH PRODUCTS

Trillium Health Products
655 South Orcas, Suite 220
Seattle, WA 98108
(206) 762-3306

JOURNALS / MAGAZINES

American Fitness Magazine
15250 Ventura Blvd., Suite 310
Sherman Oaks, CA 91403
Peg Jordan, RN, Editor
(800) 445-5950